DOG BREEDS

A Picture Book for People Who Like Dogs, Not Words

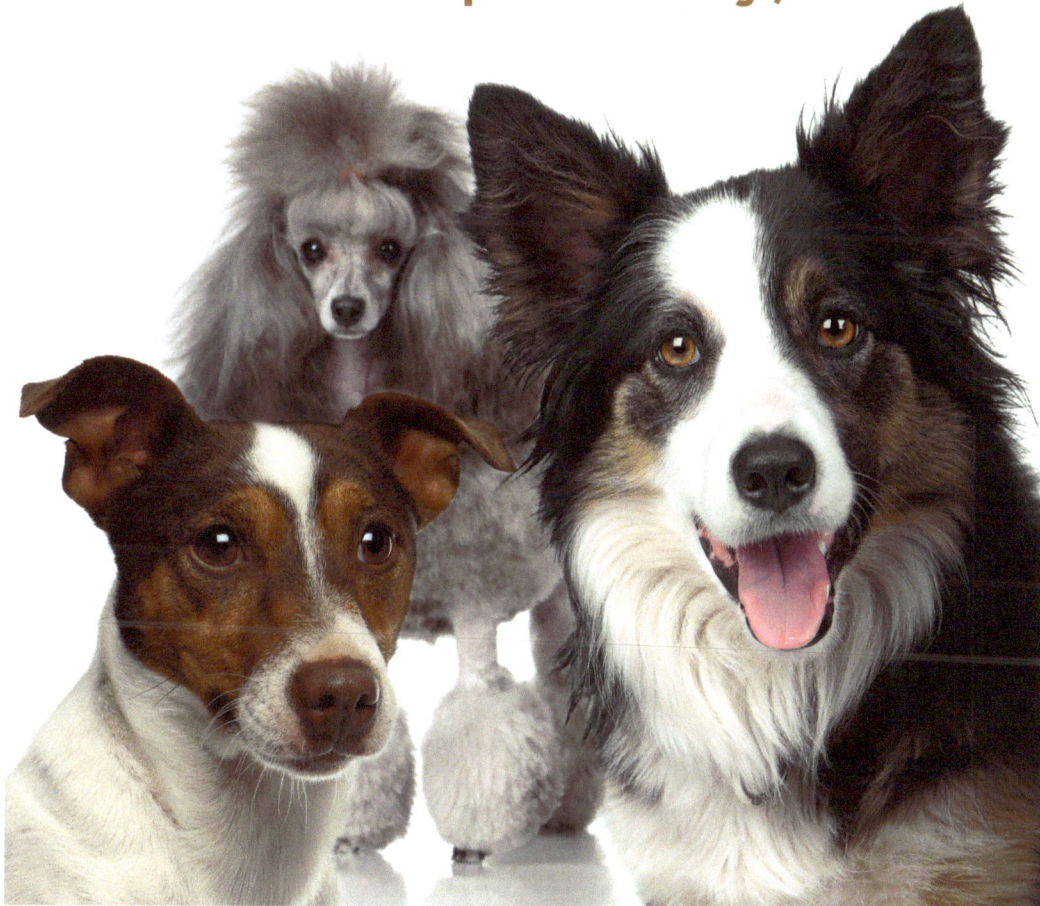

Copyright © 2020 by Lasting Happiness
ISBN: 978-1-989842-01-0

Akita

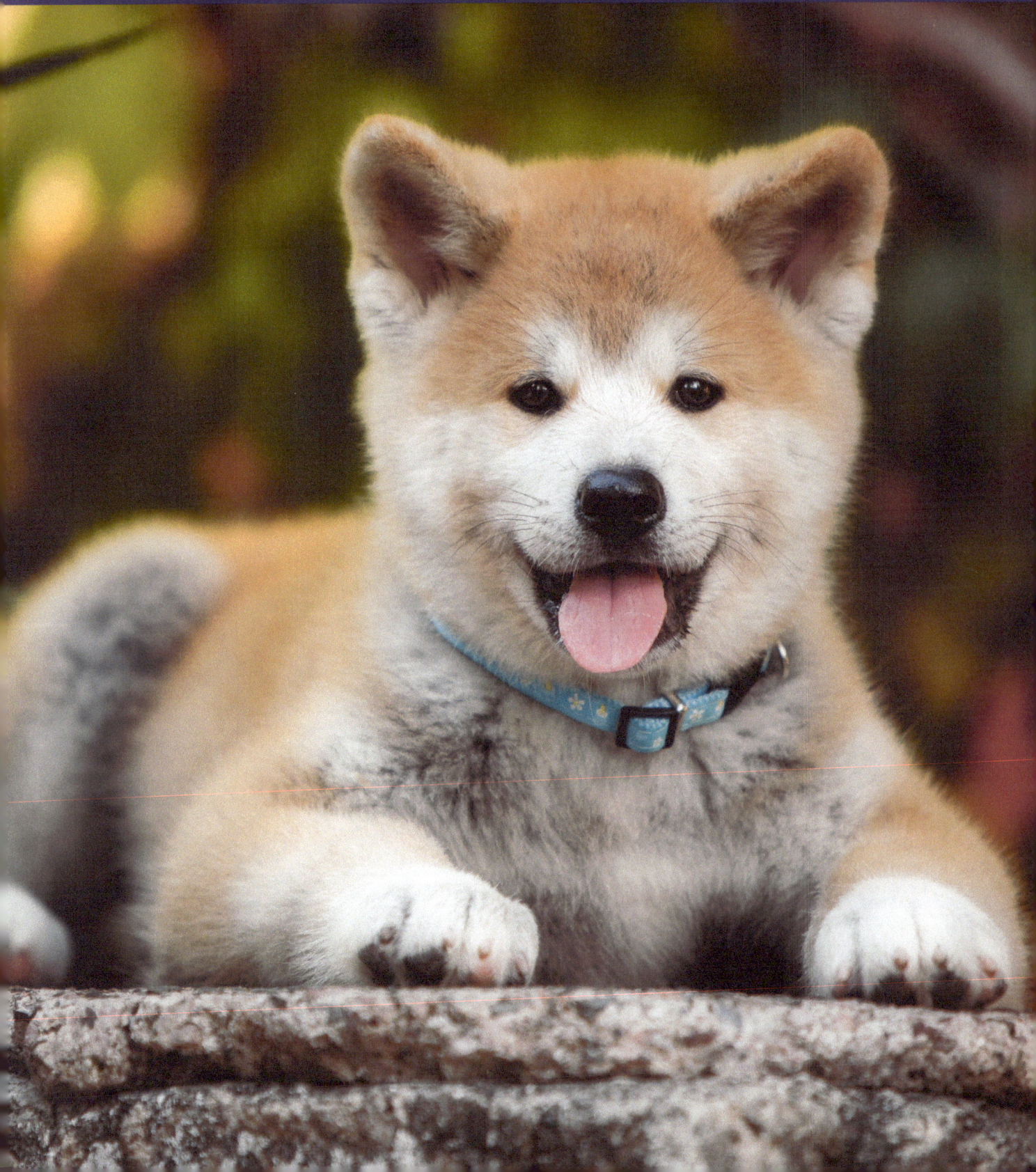

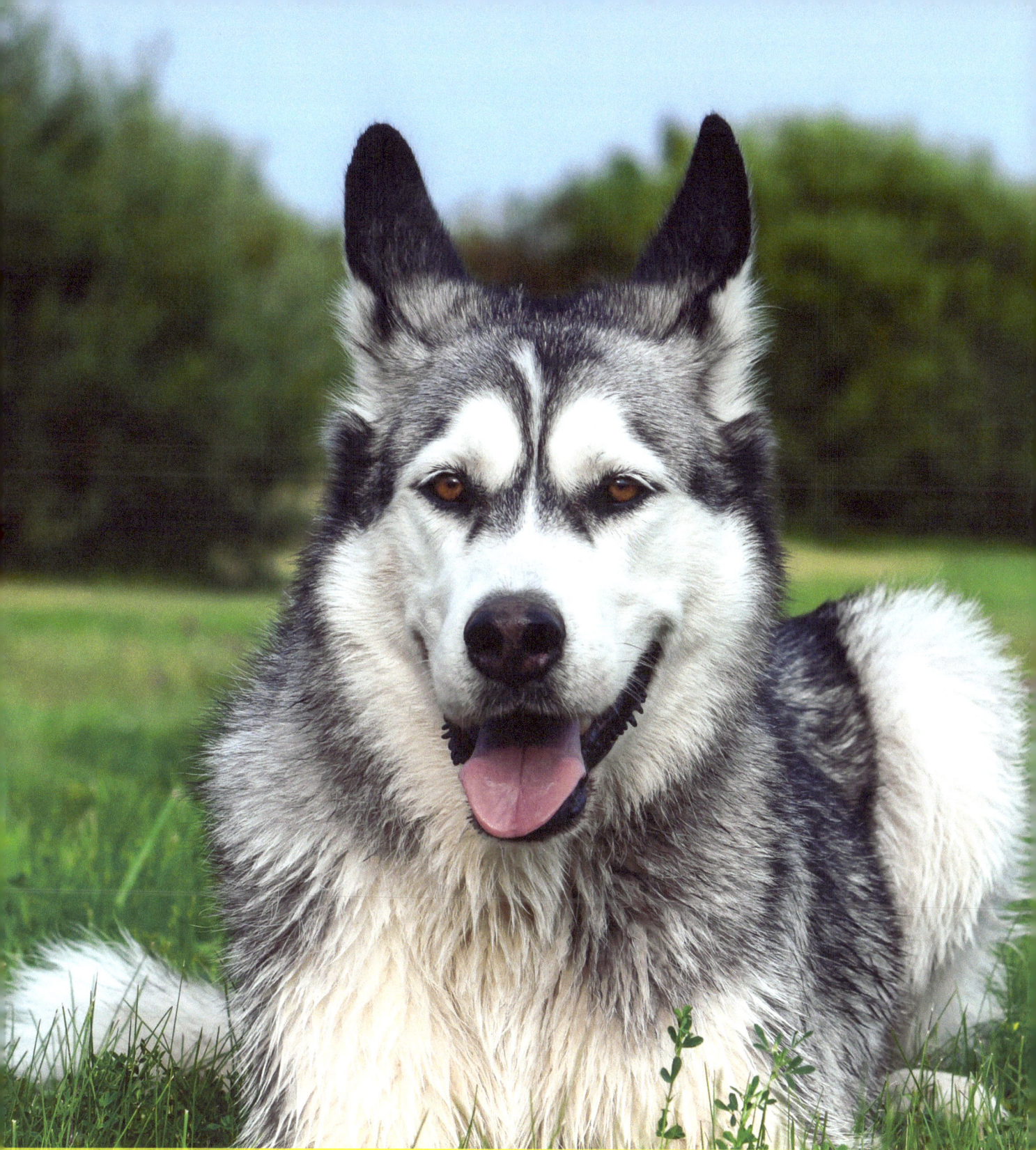

Alaskan Malamute

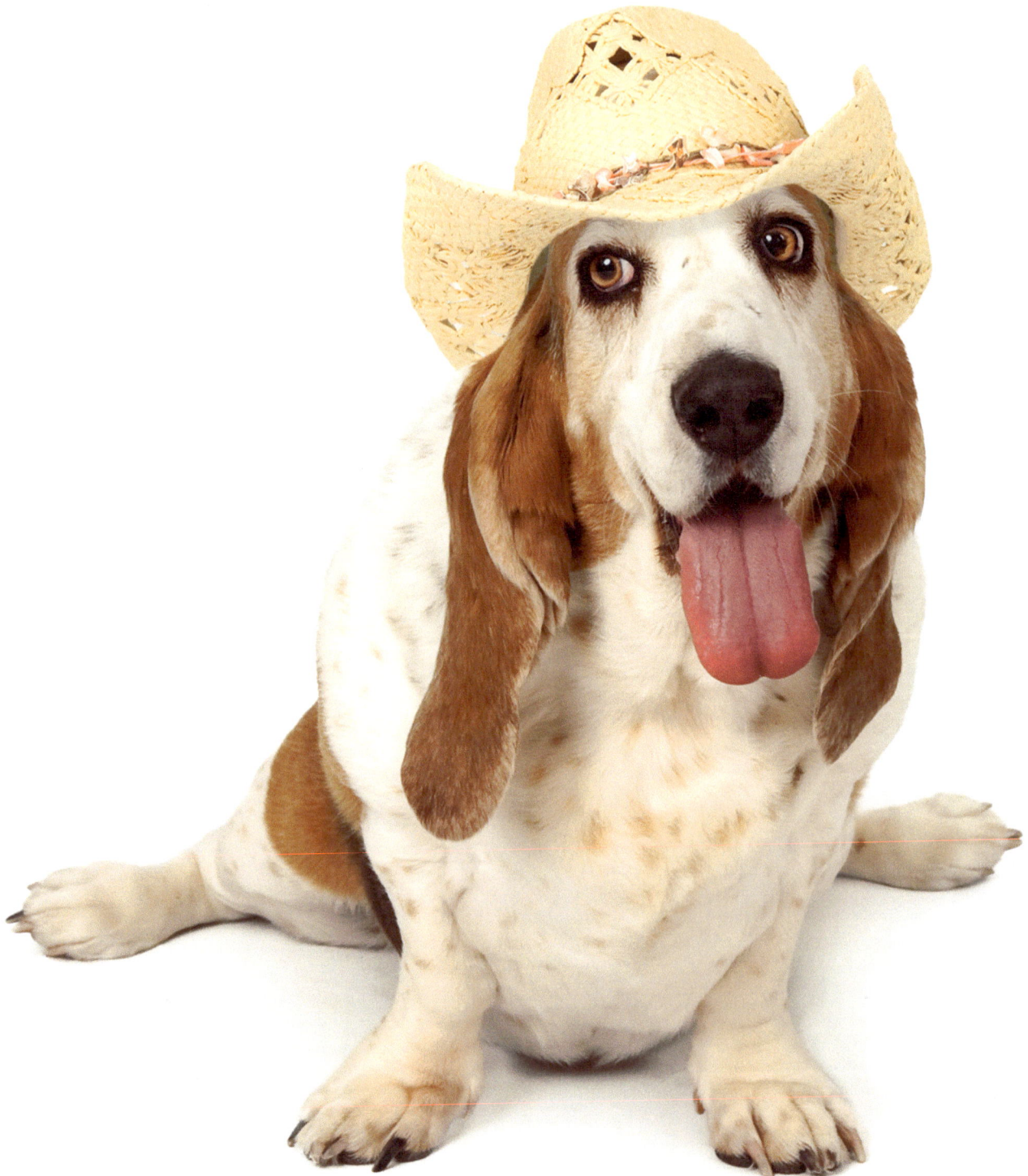

Basset Hound

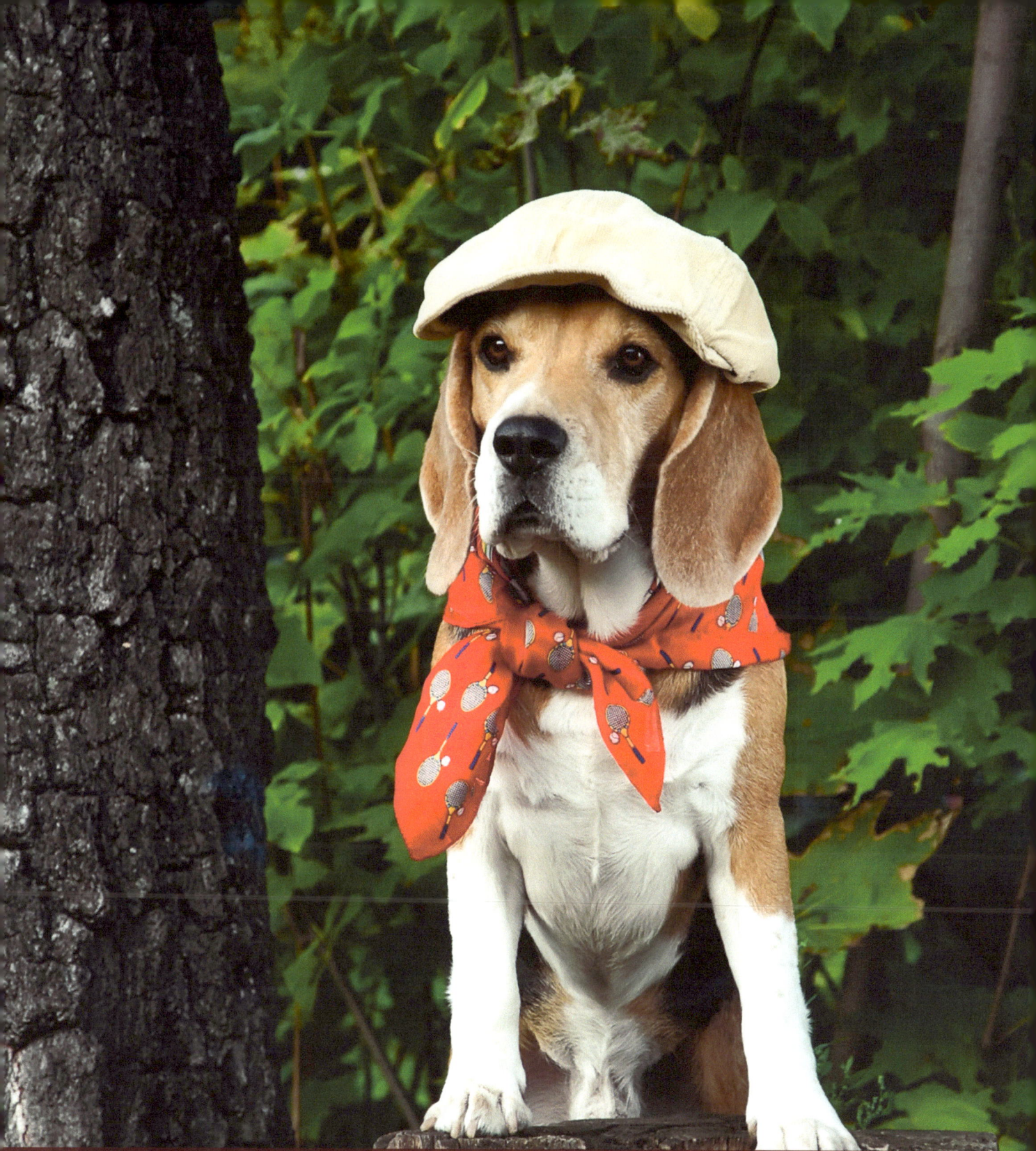

Beagle

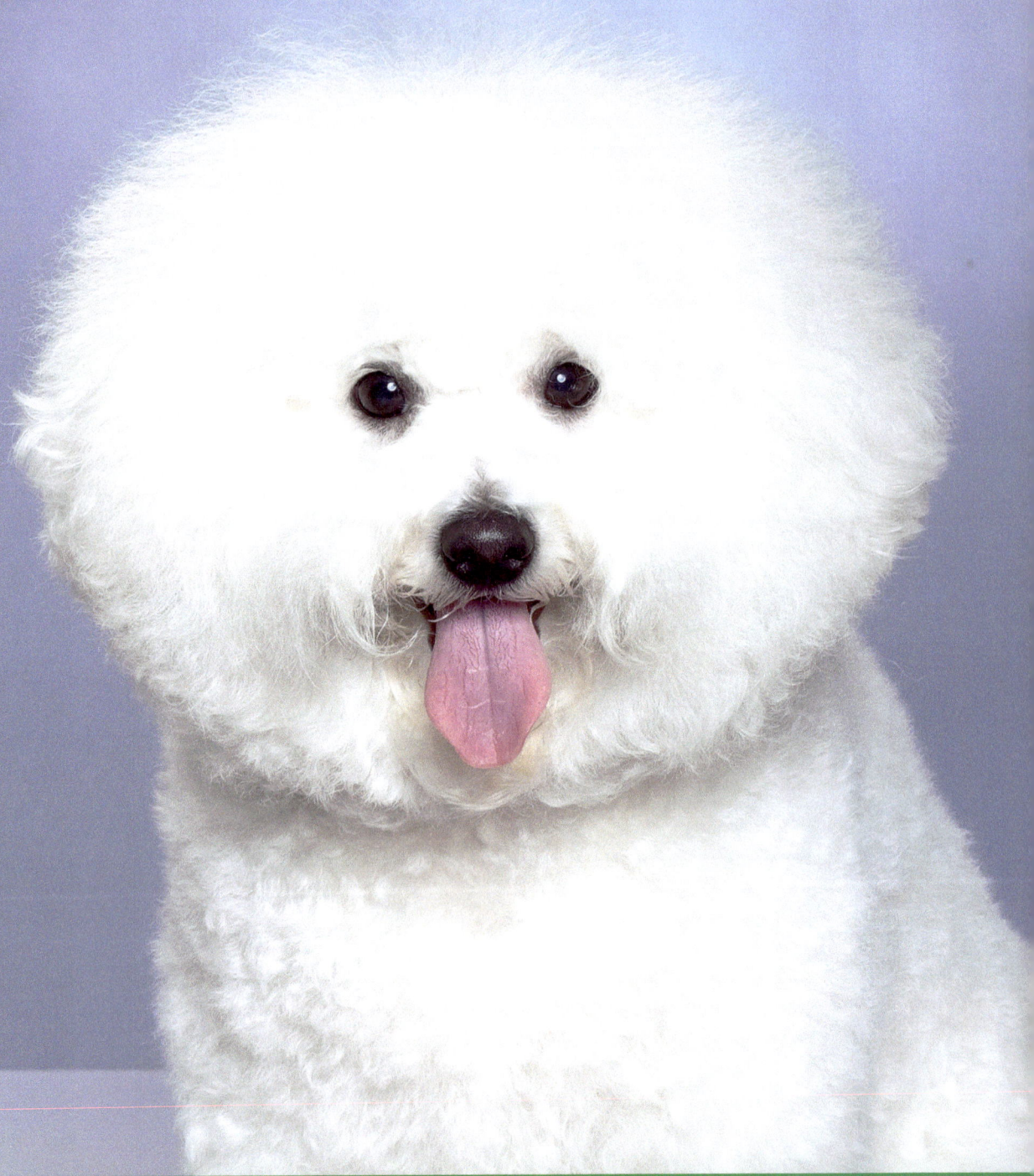

Bichon
Frise

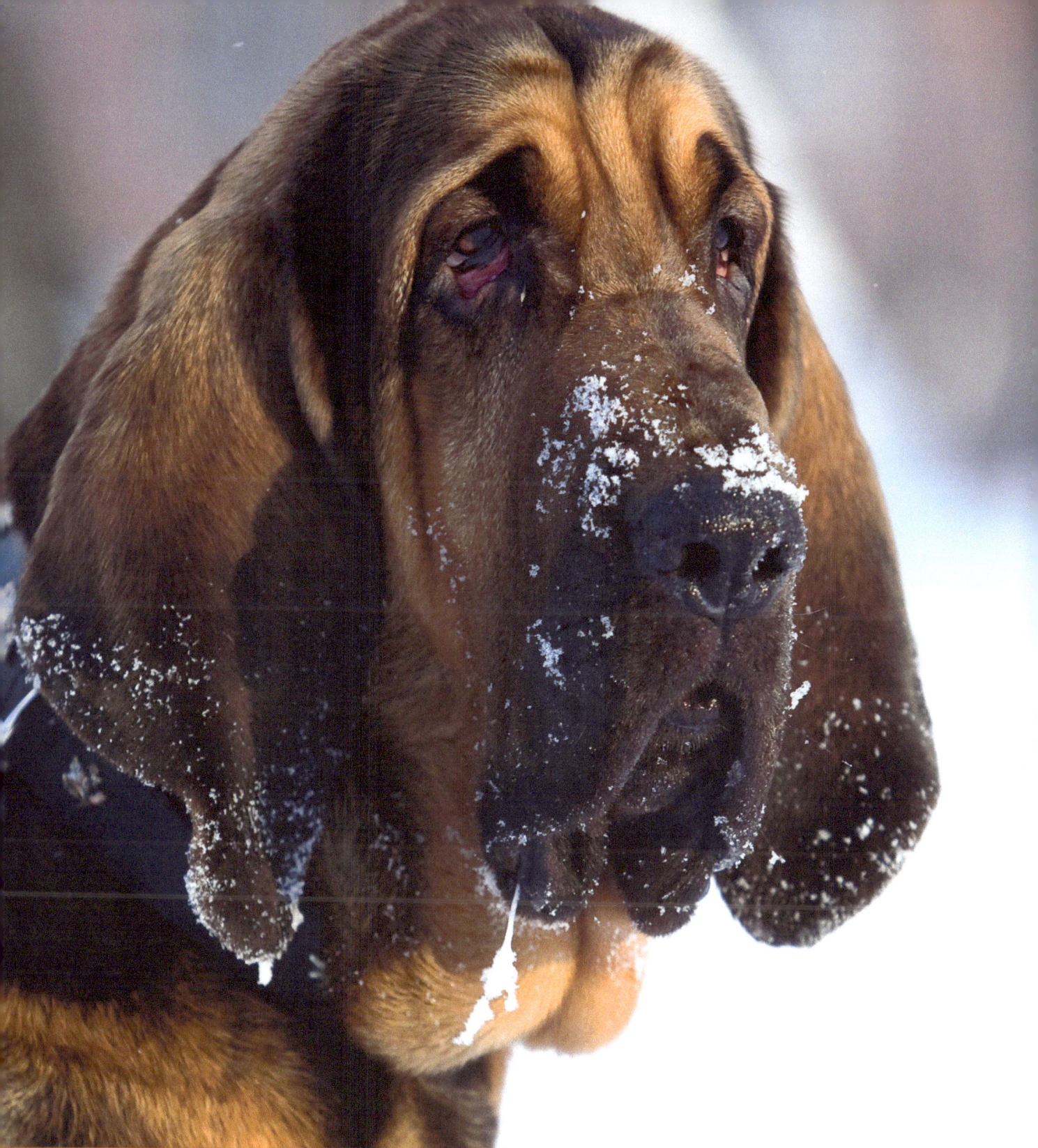

Bloodhound

Border Collie

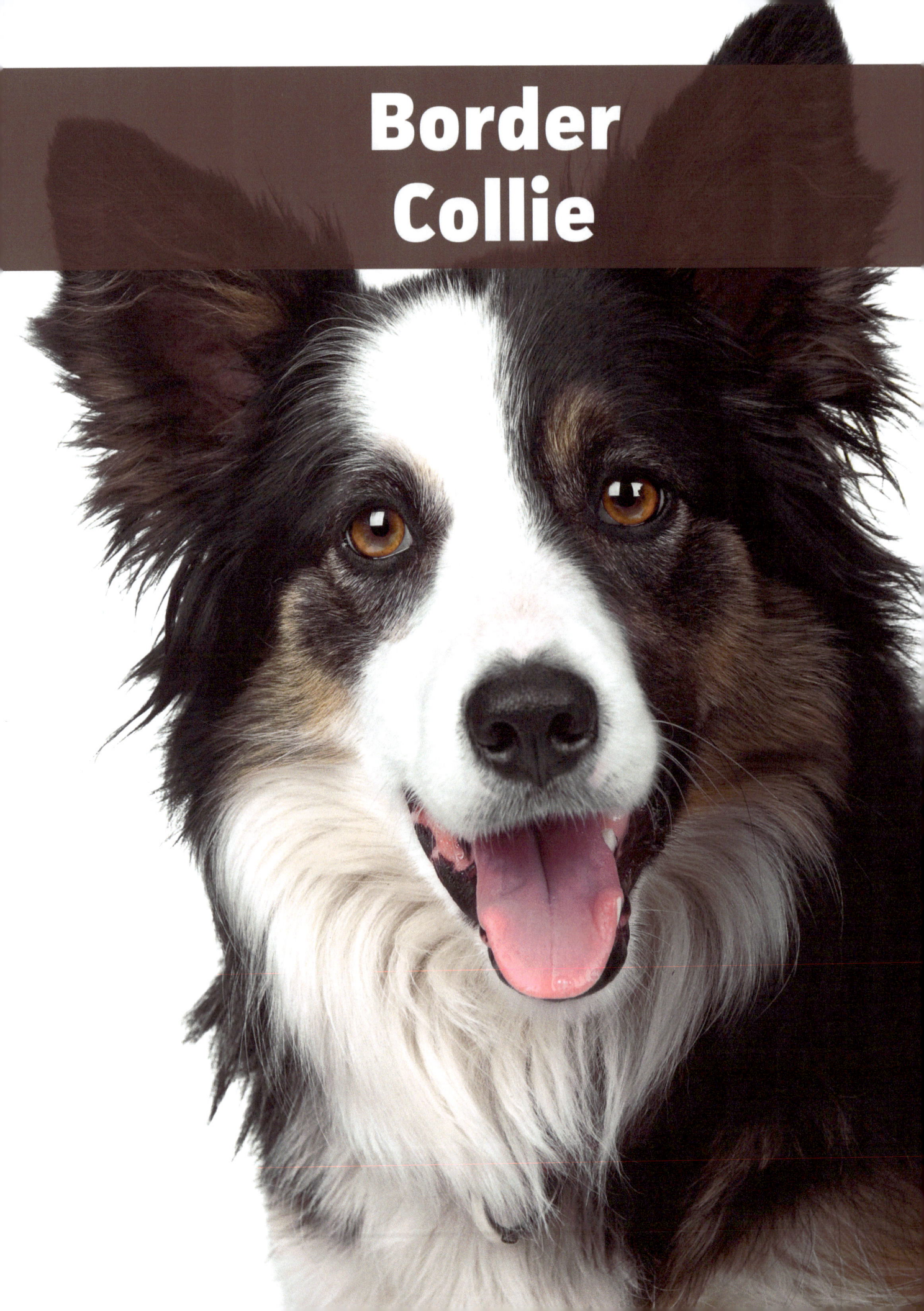

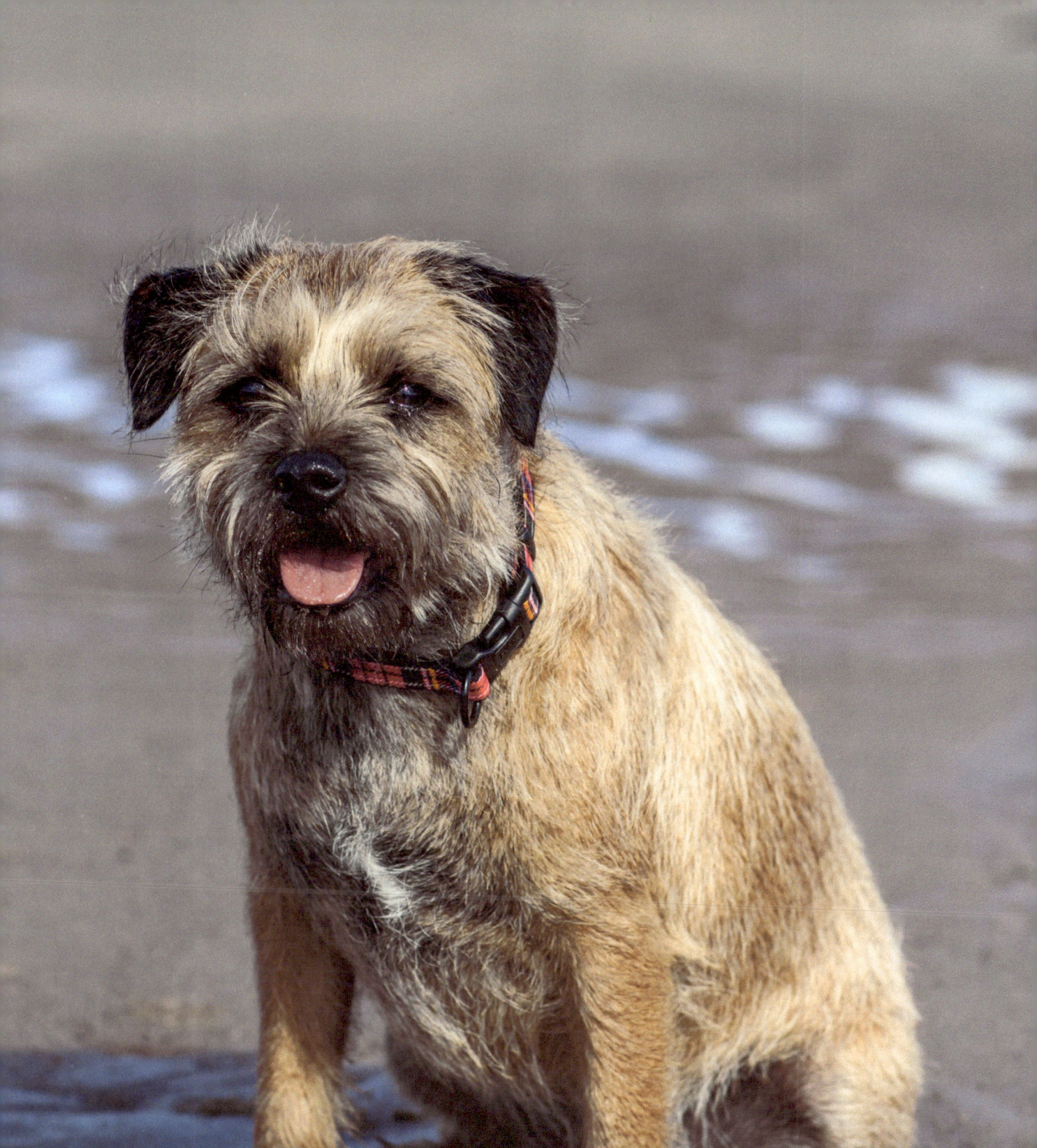

Border Terrier

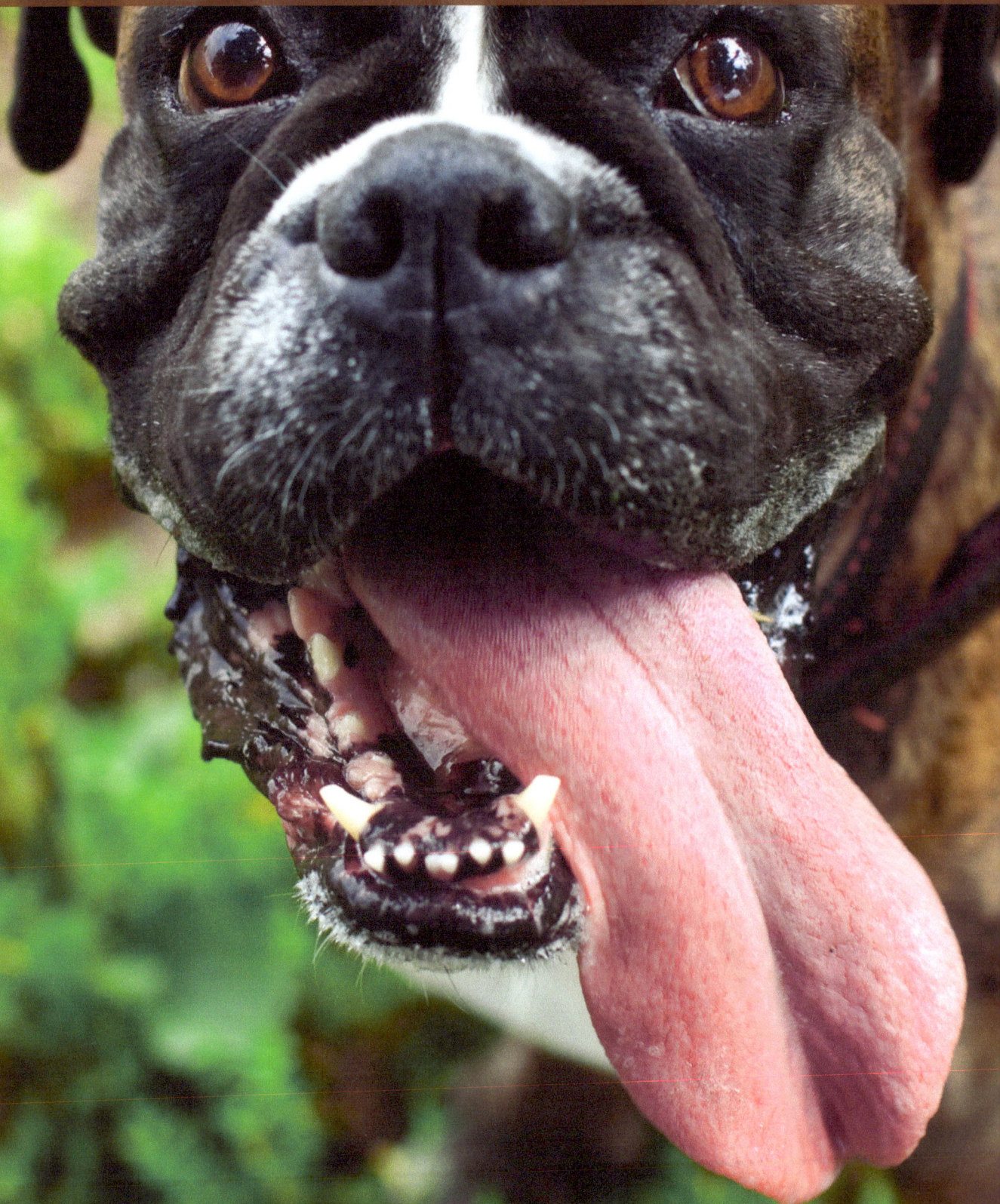

Boxer

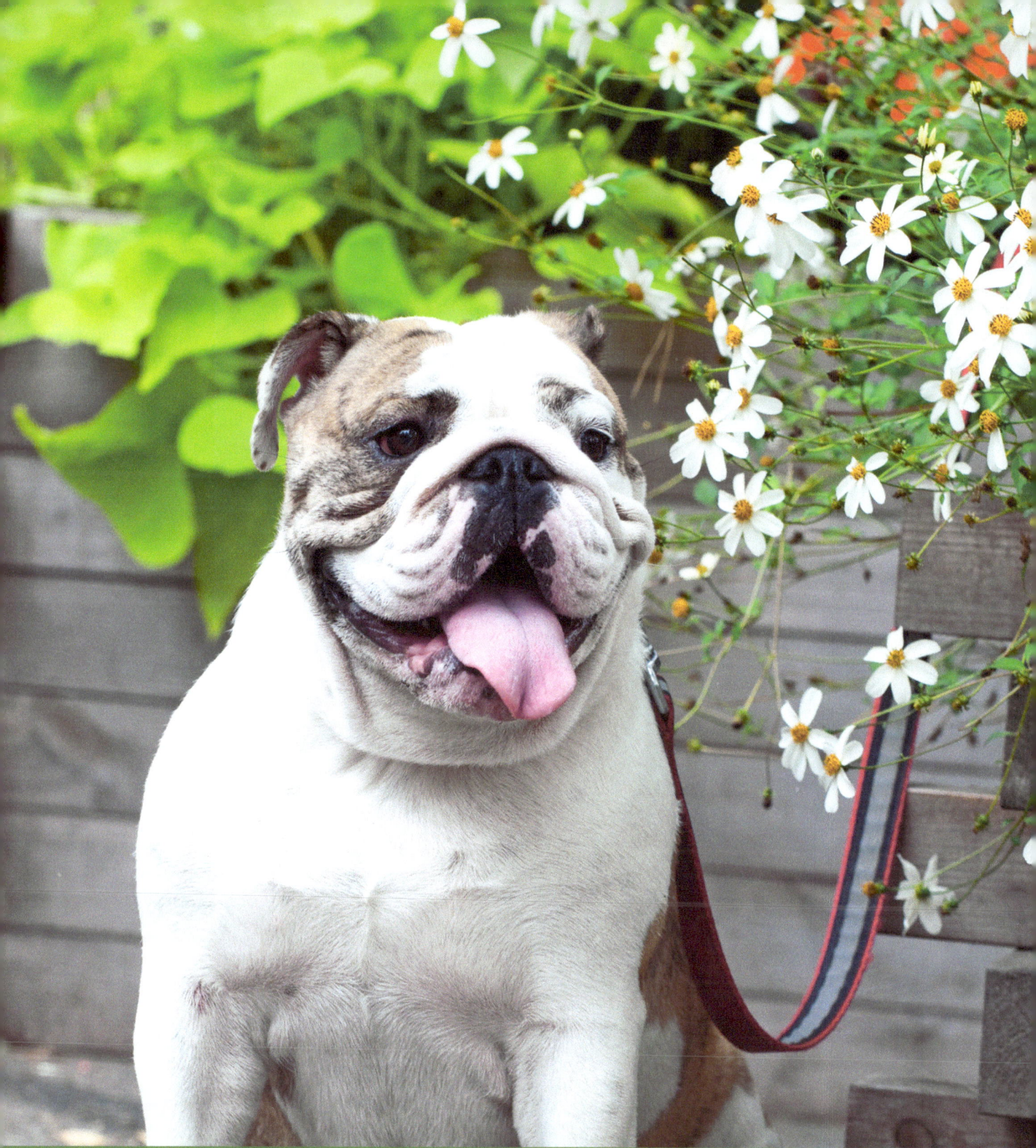

British Bulldog

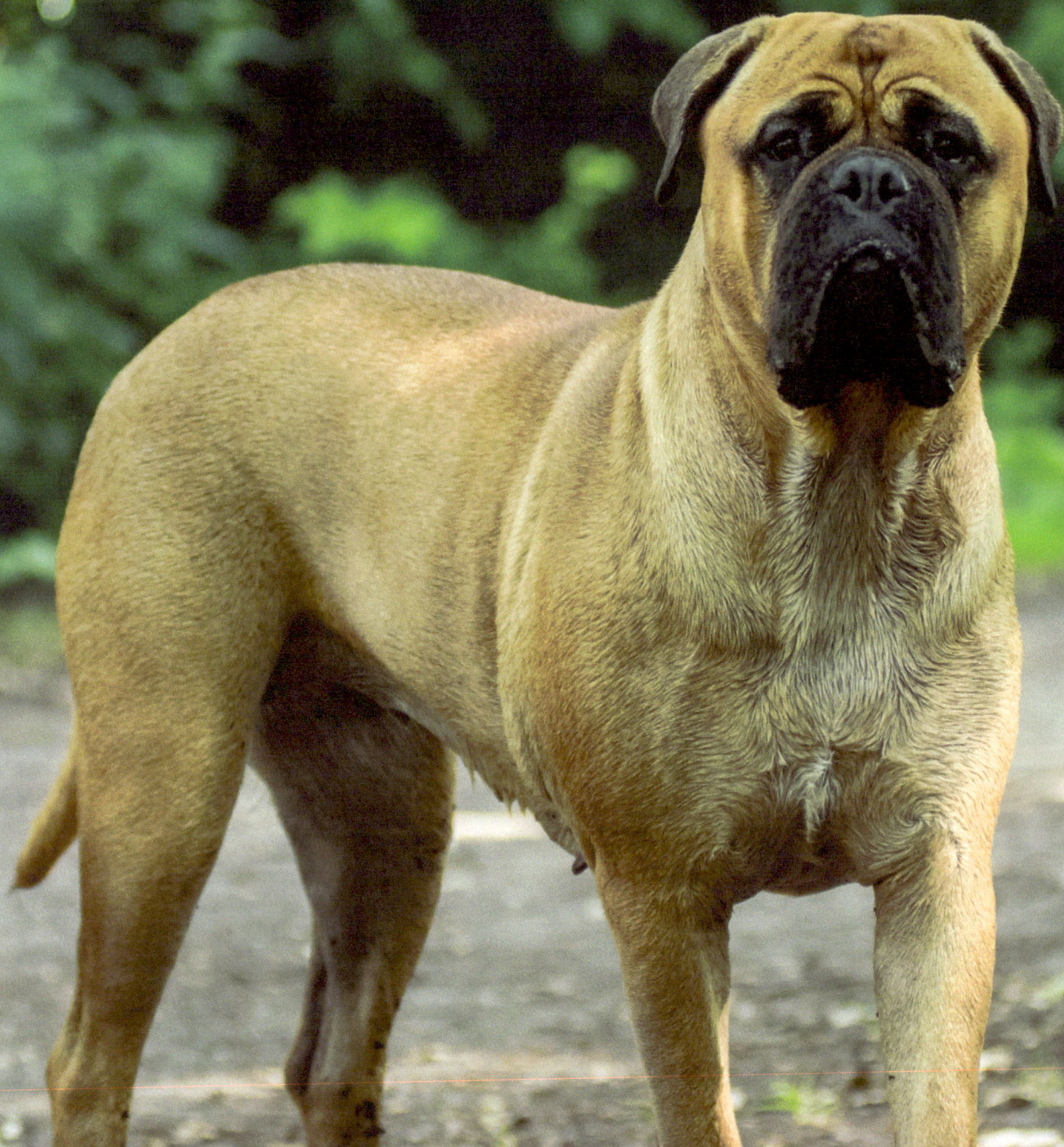

Bullmastiff

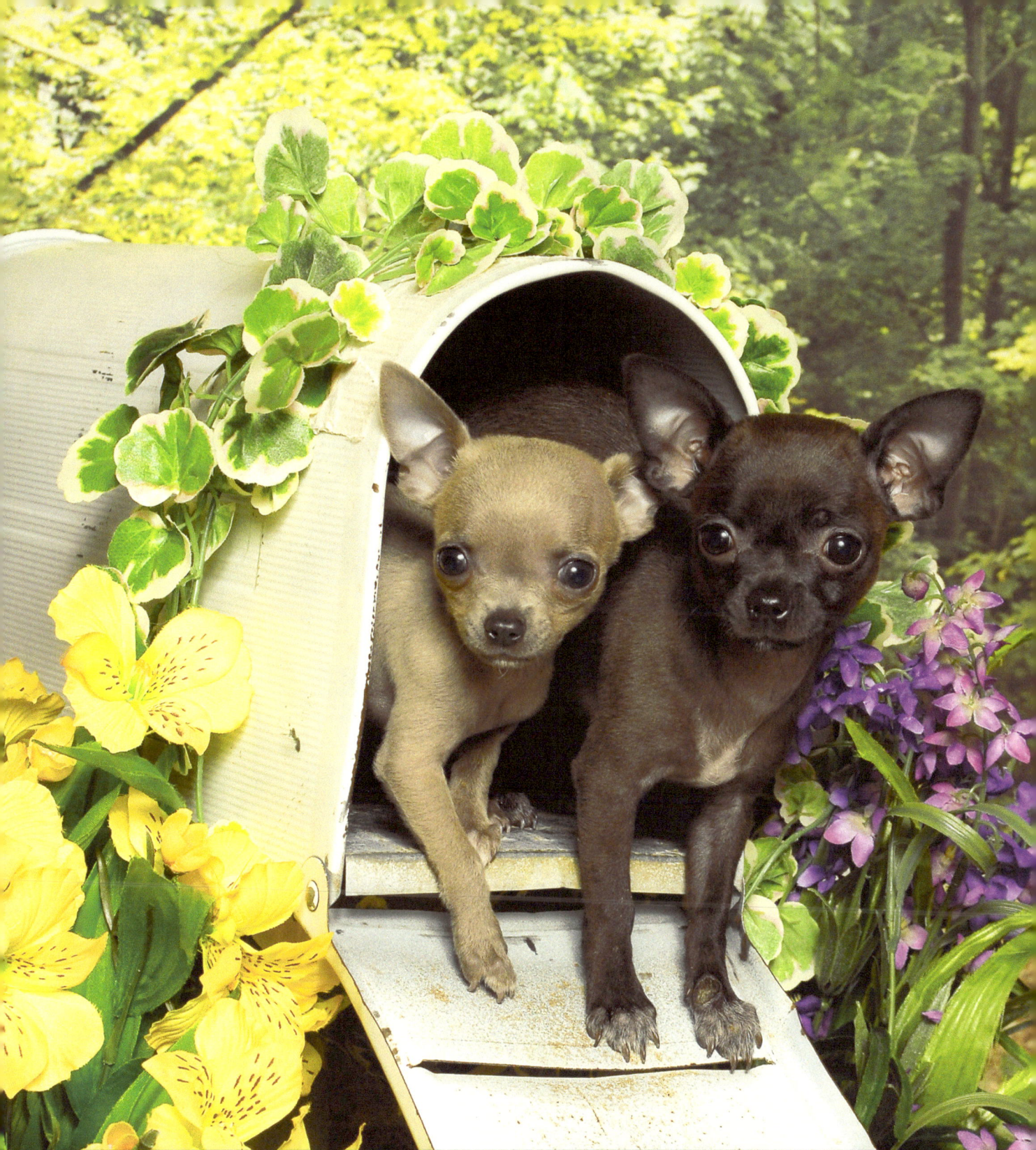

Chihuahua

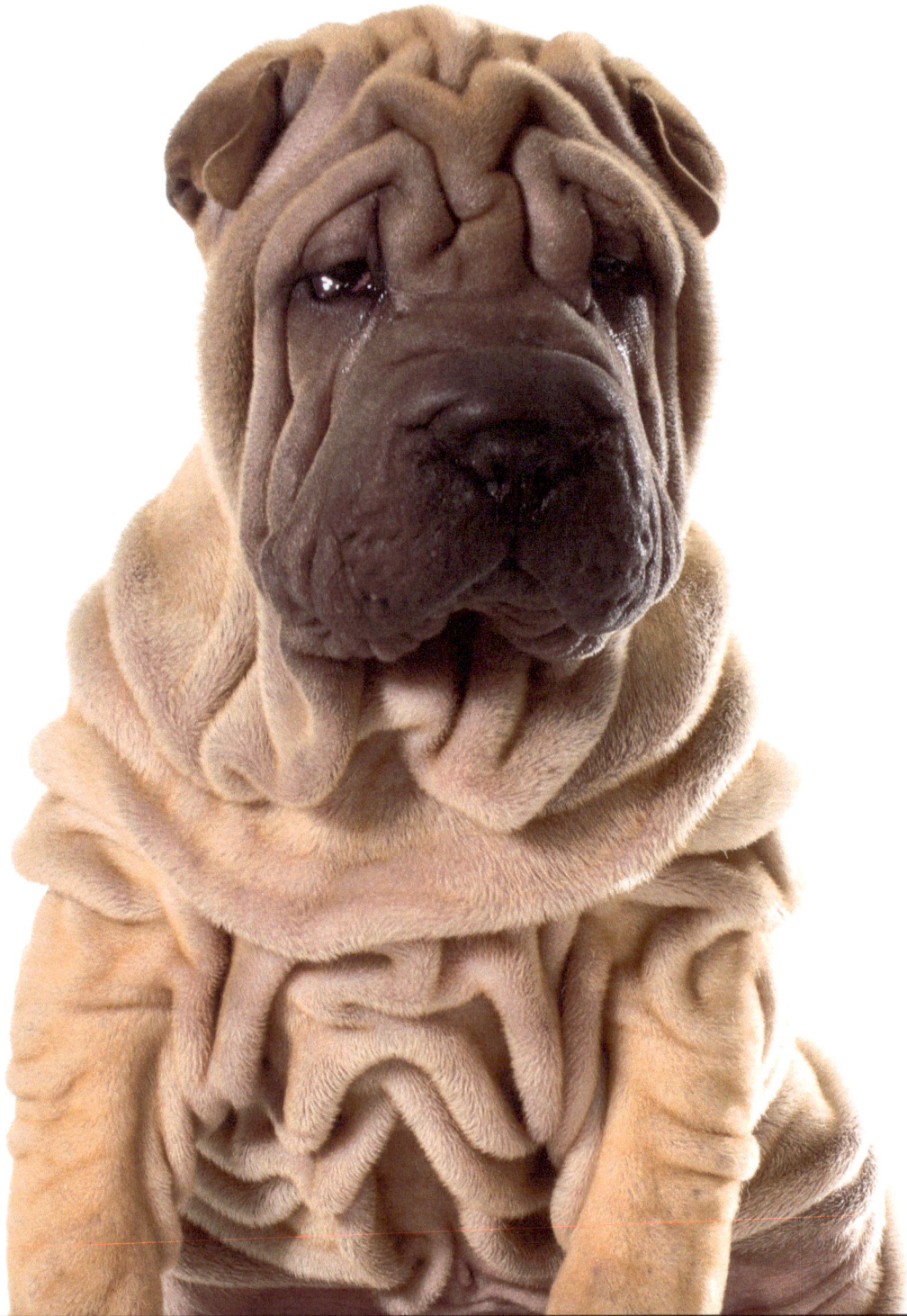

Chinese Shar-Pei

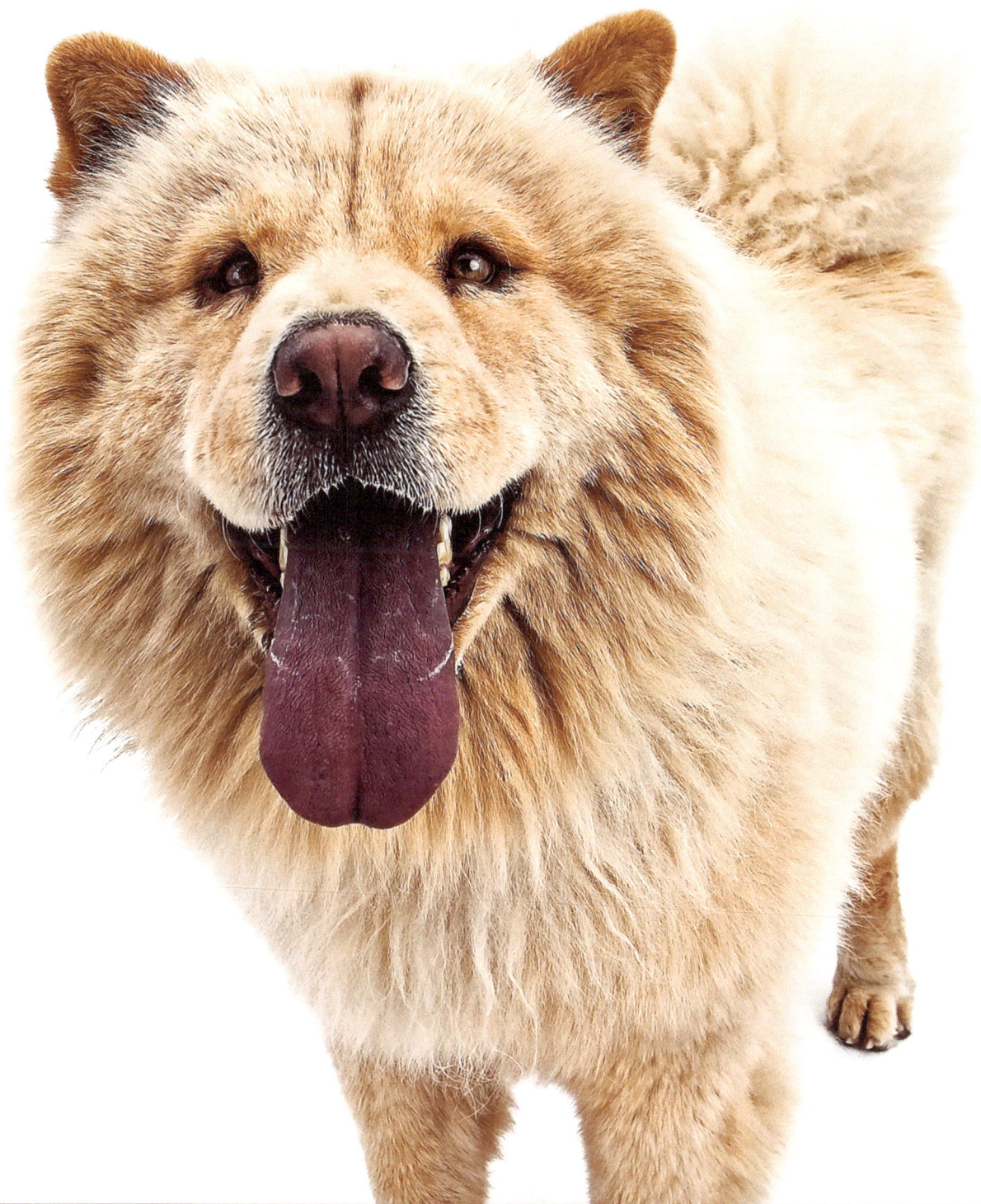

Chow Chow

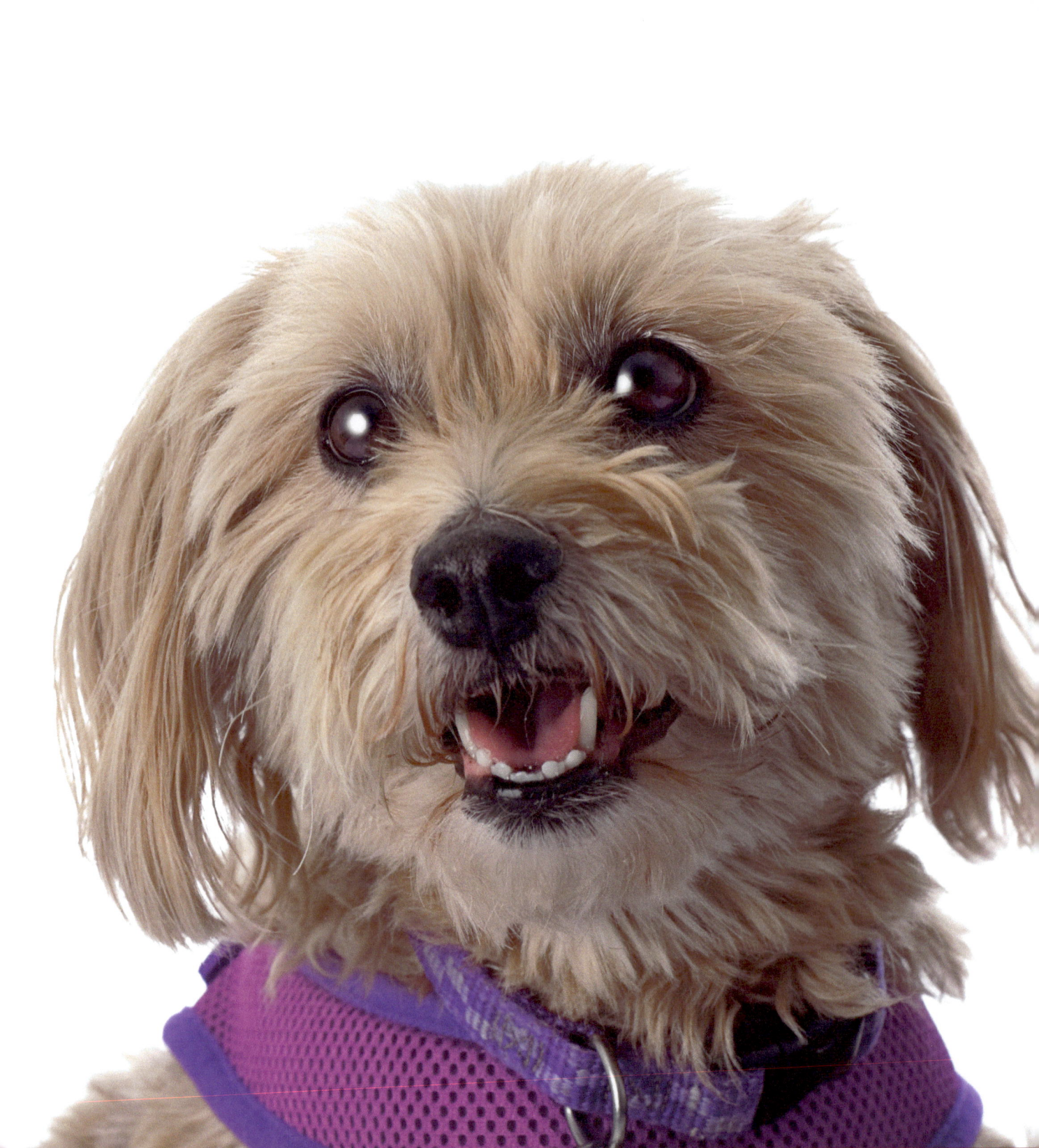

Cockapoo

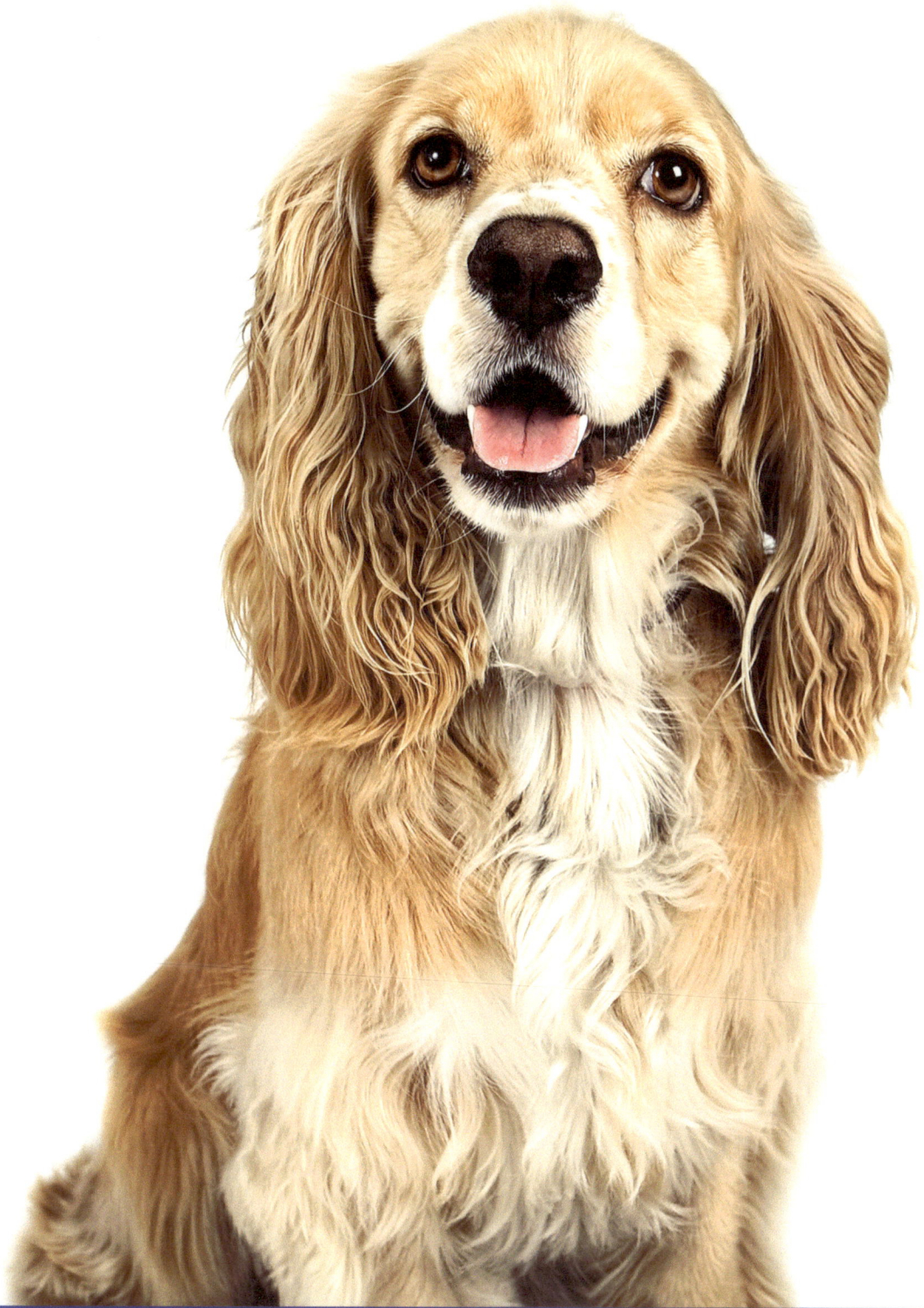

Cocker Spaniel

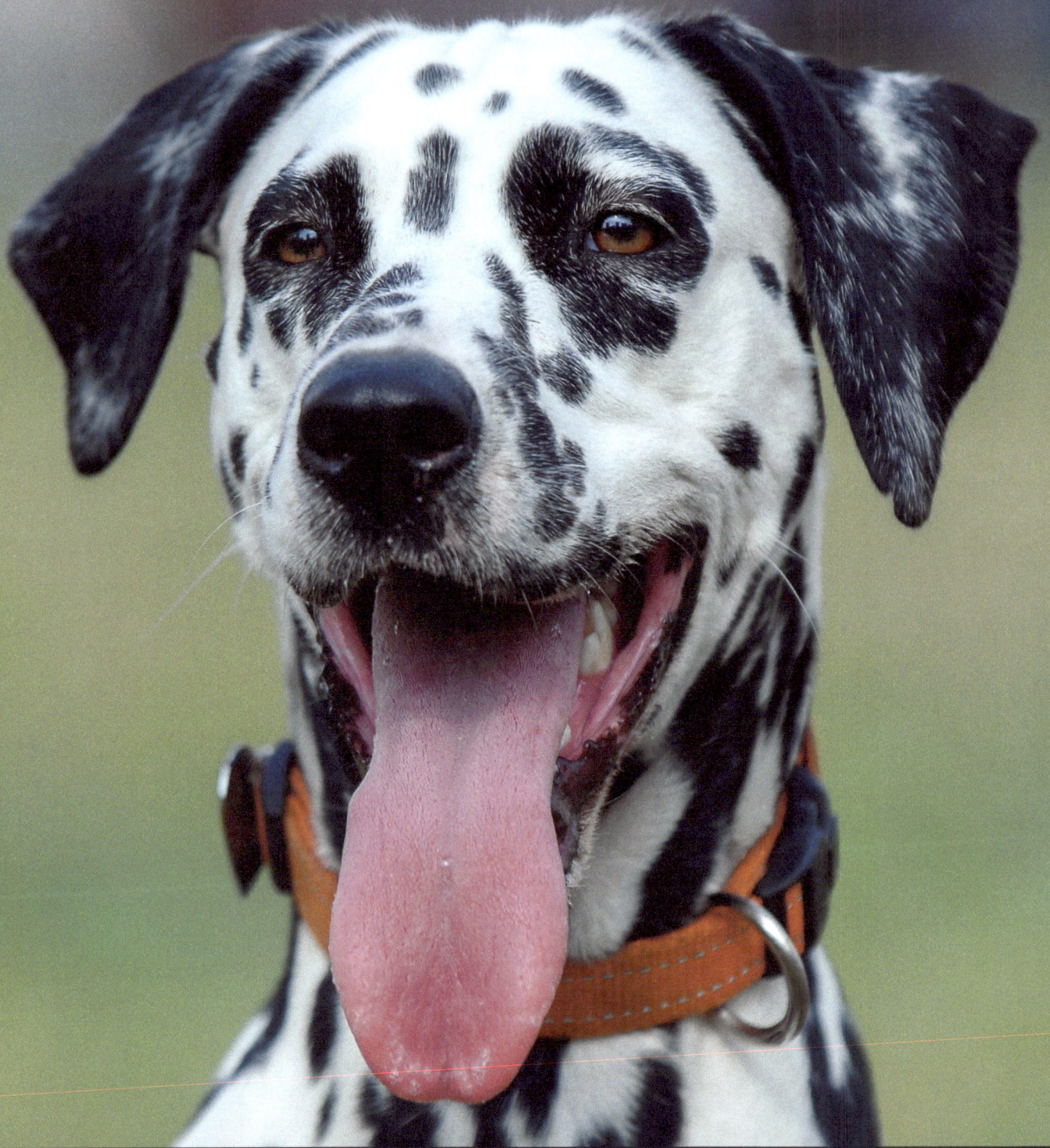

Dalmation

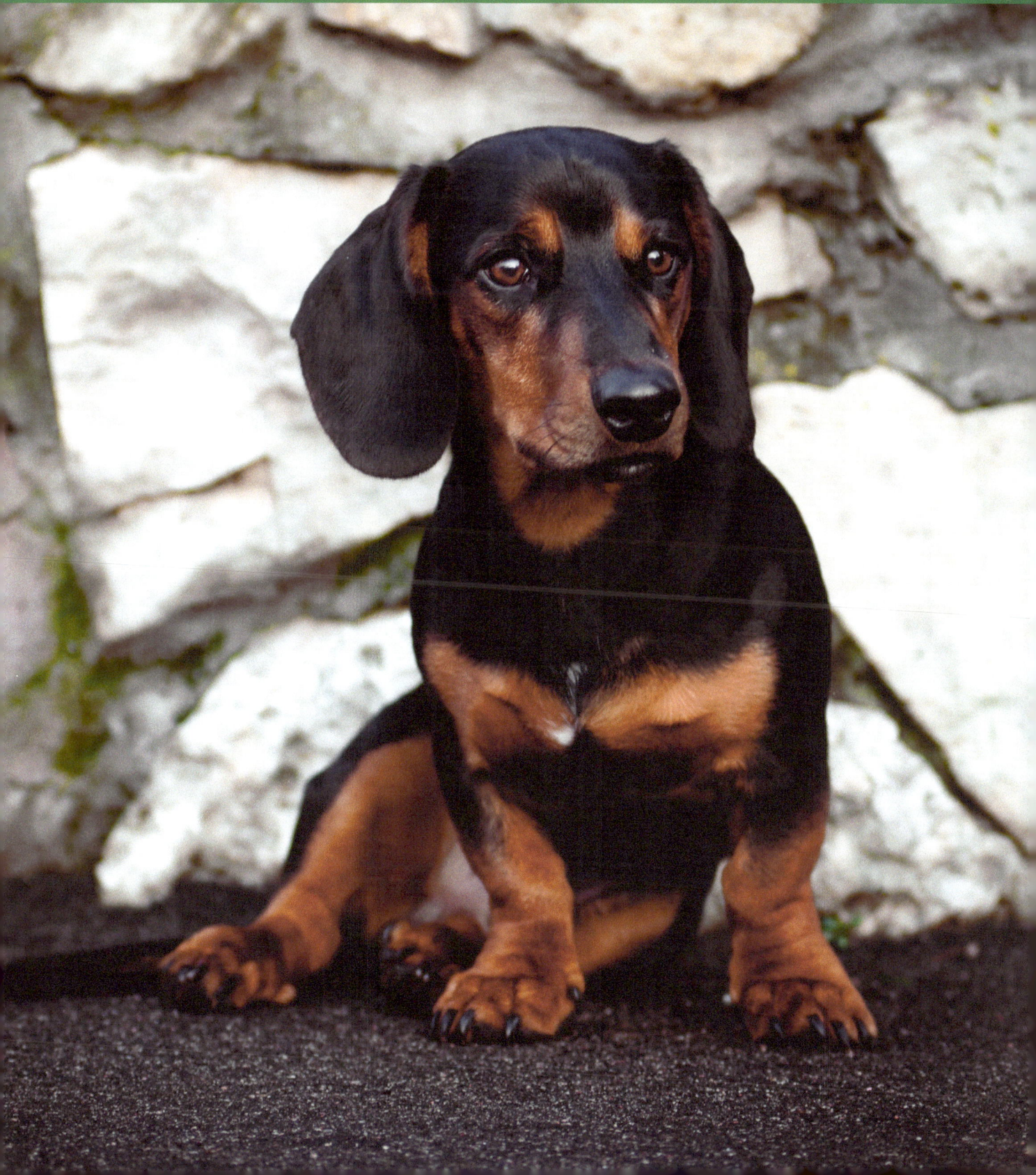

Daschund

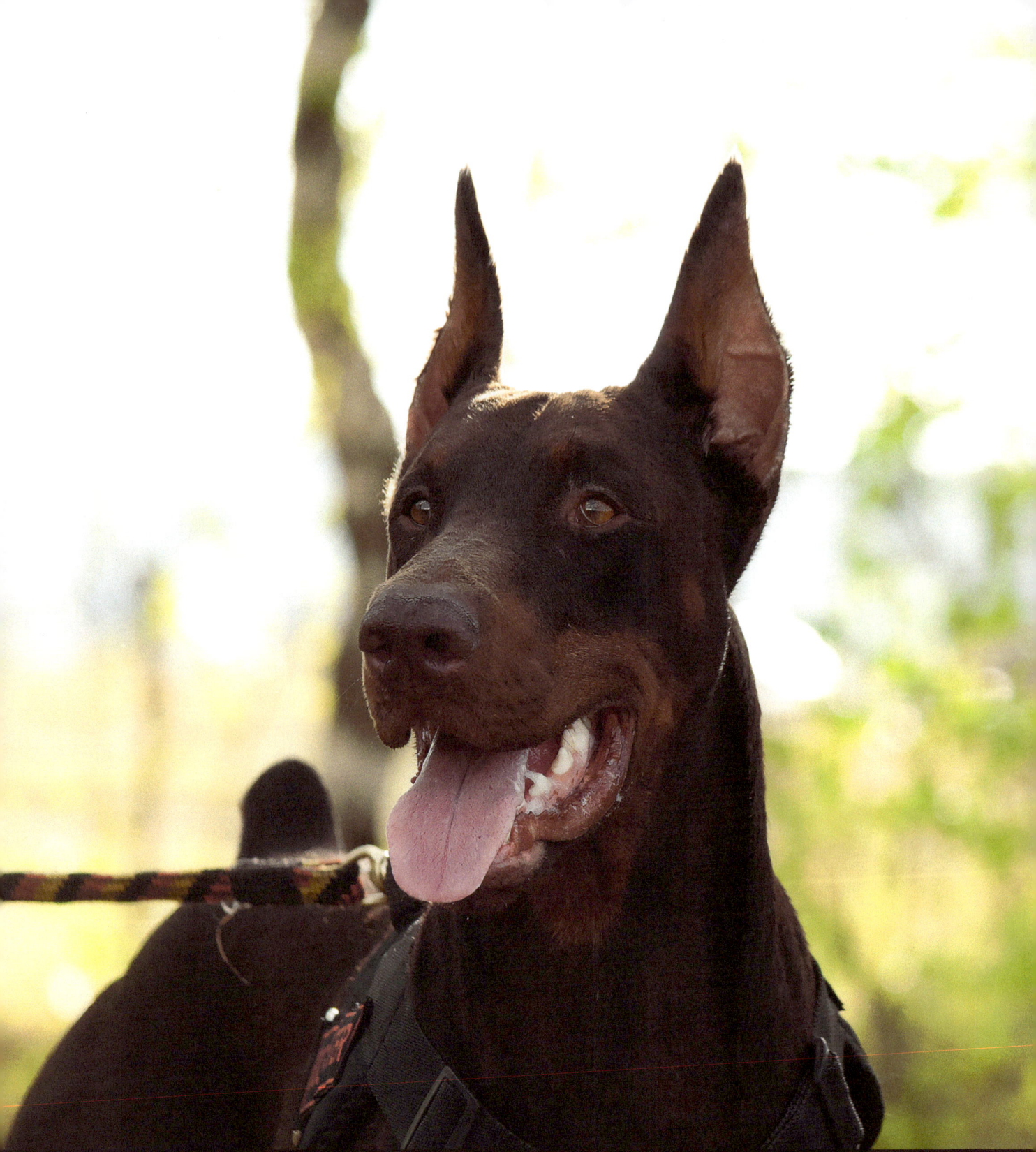

Doberman Pinscher

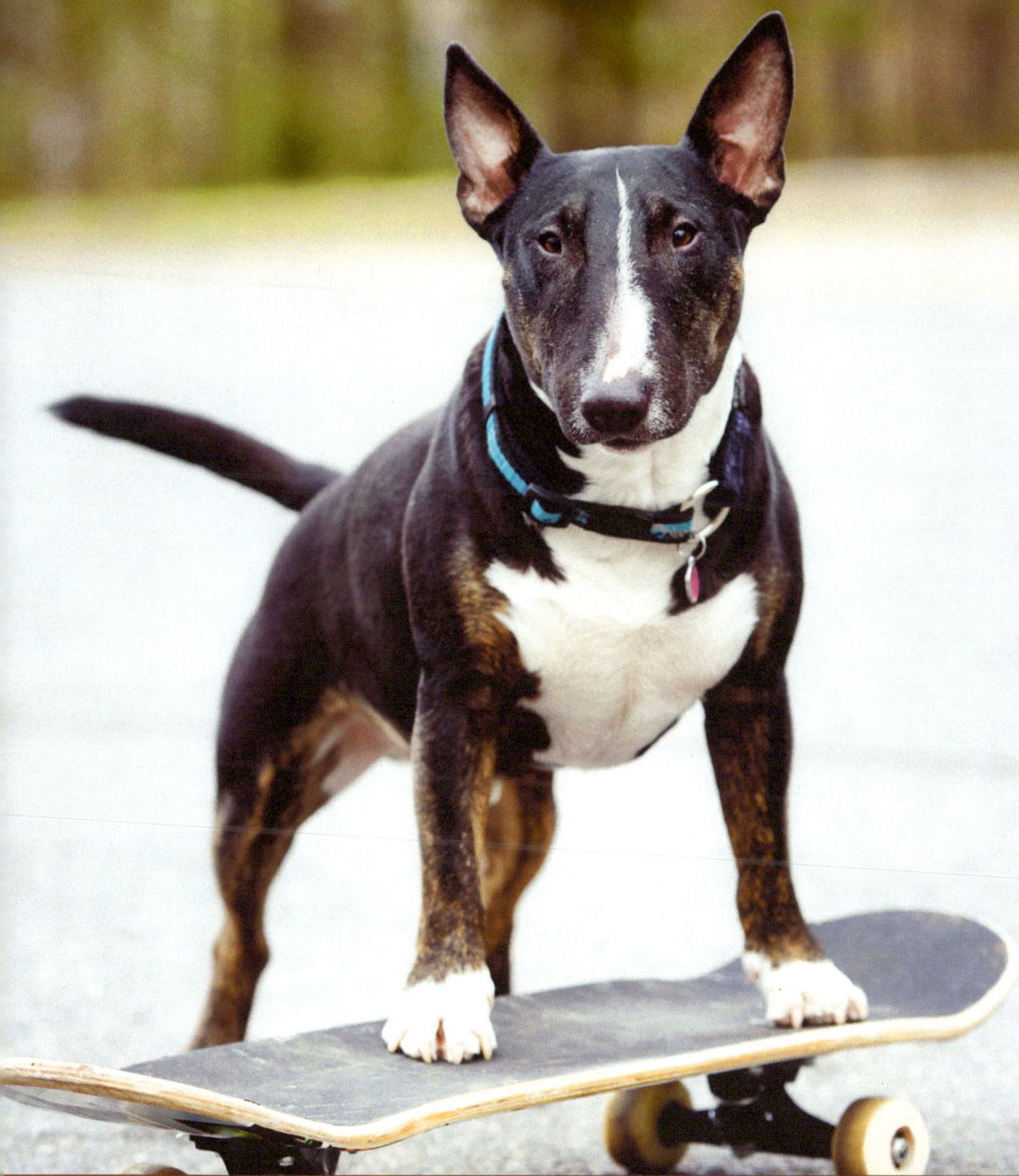

English
Bull Terrier

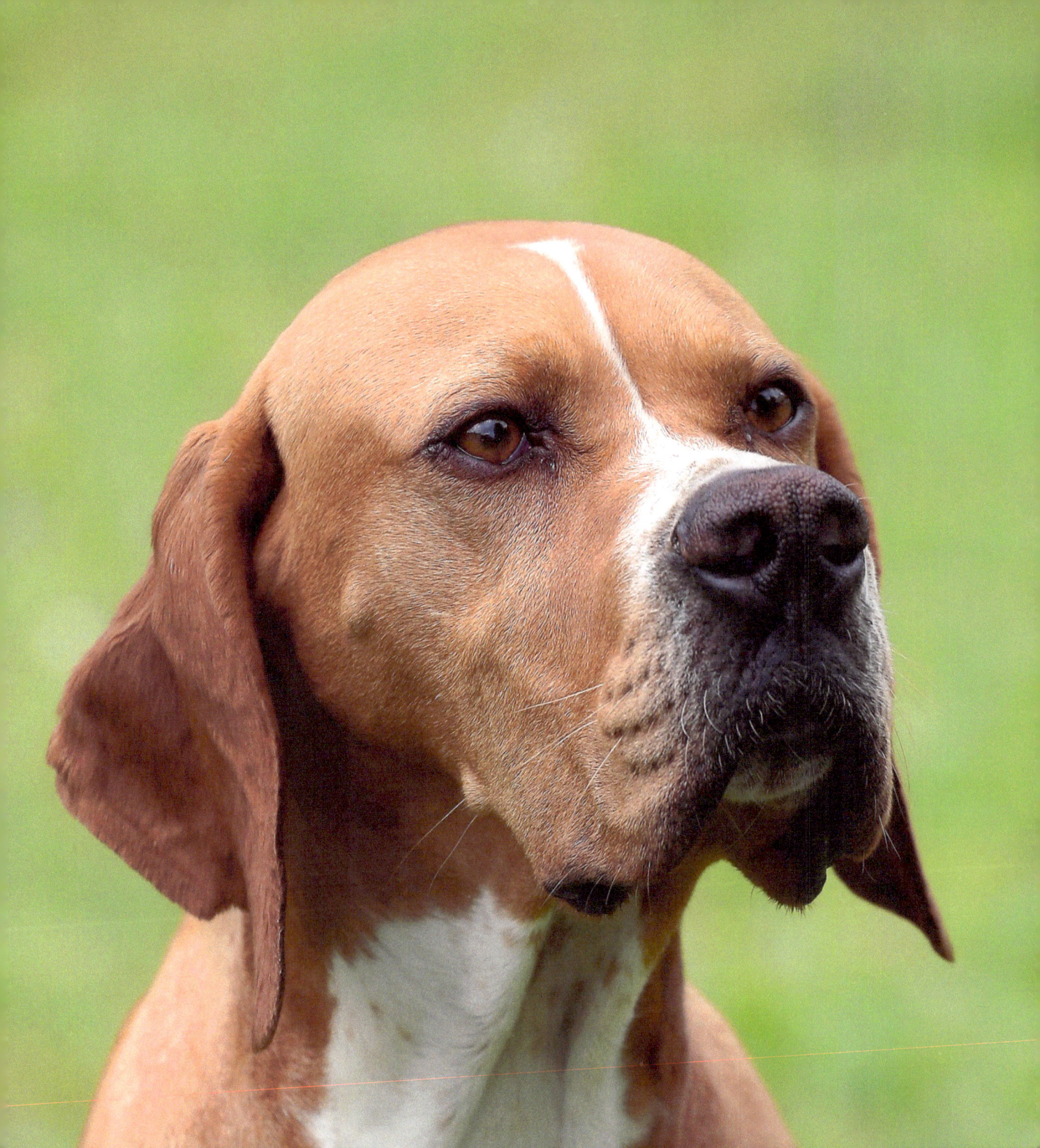

English Pointer

English Setter

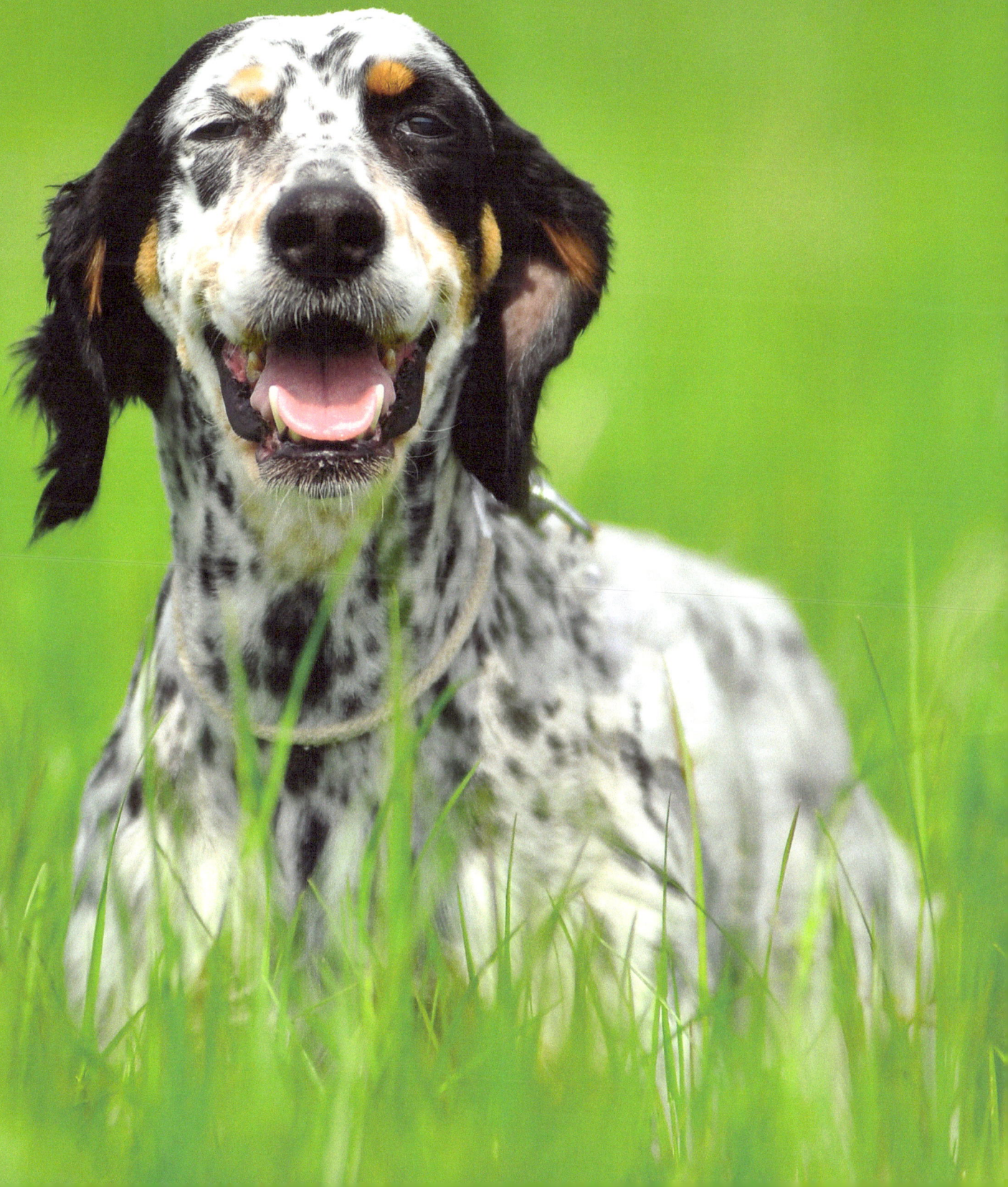

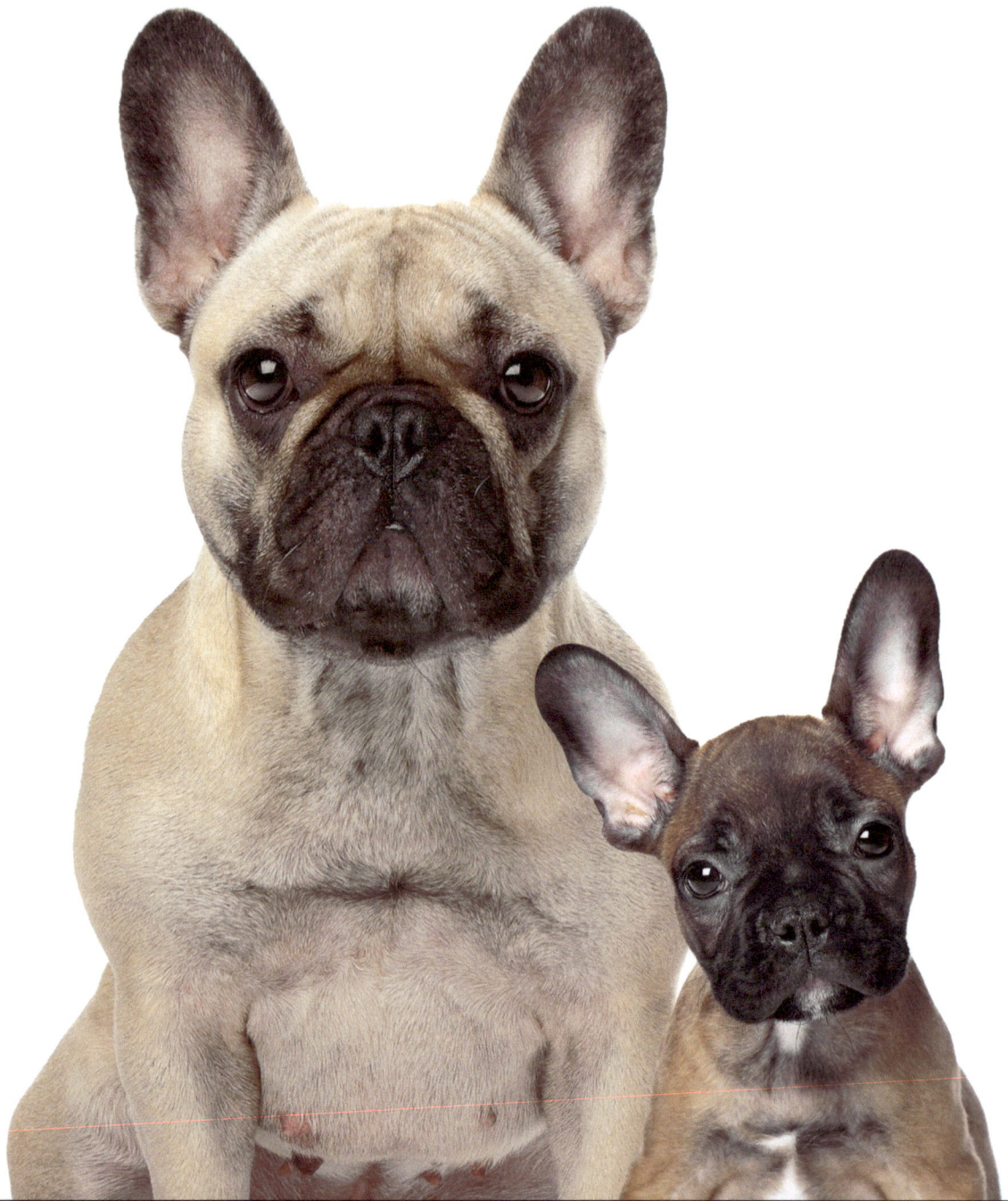

French Bulldog

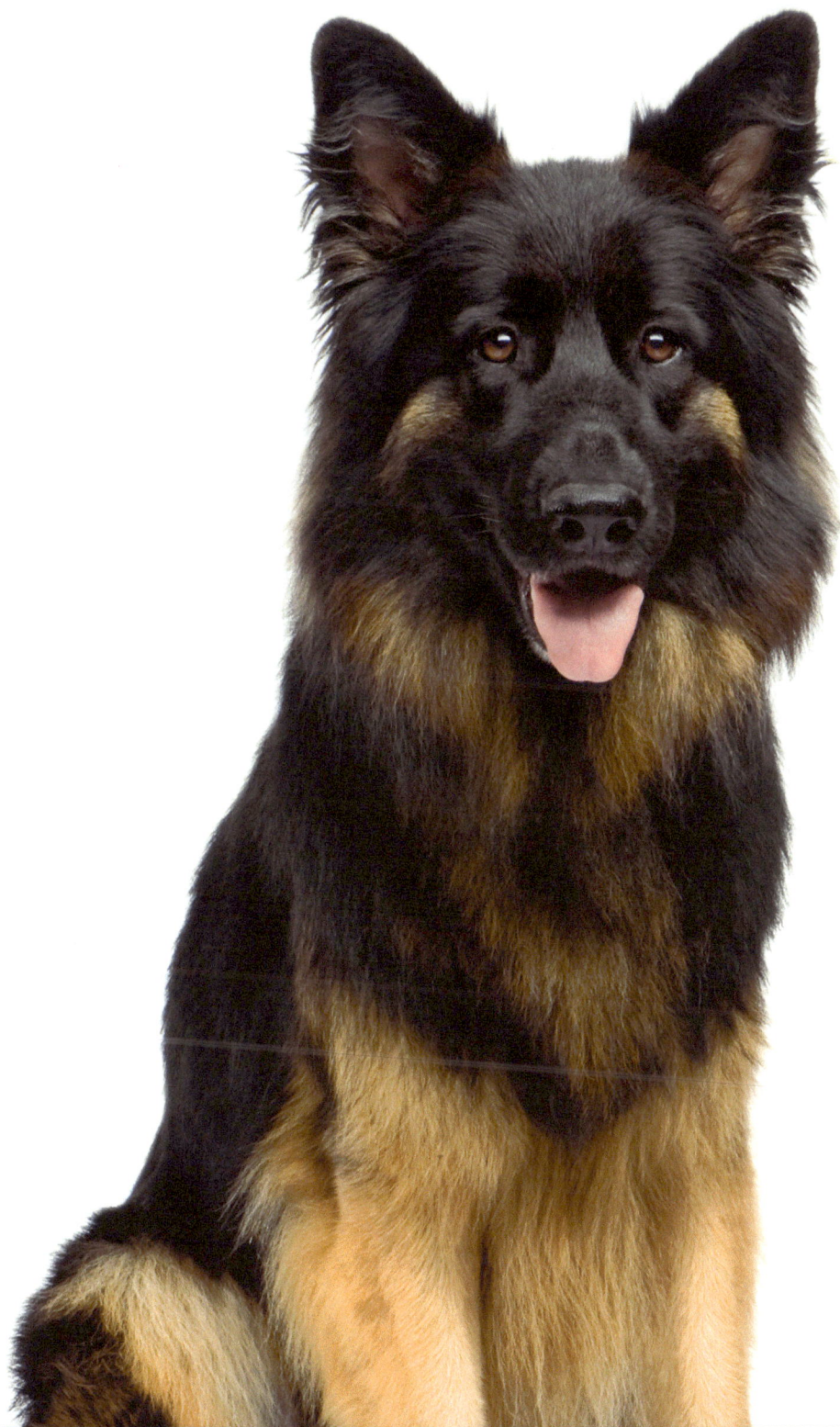

German Shepherd

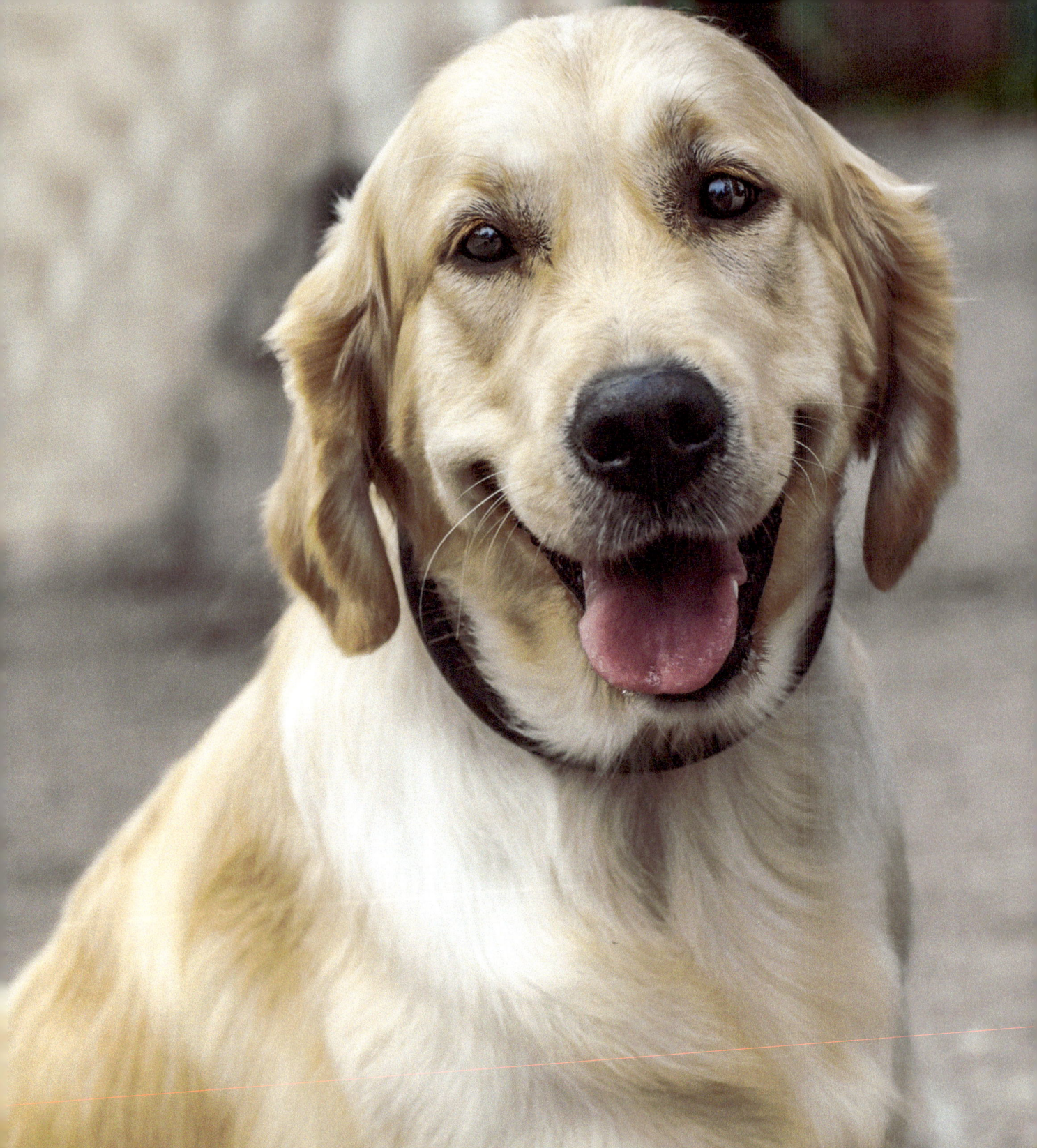

Golden Retriever

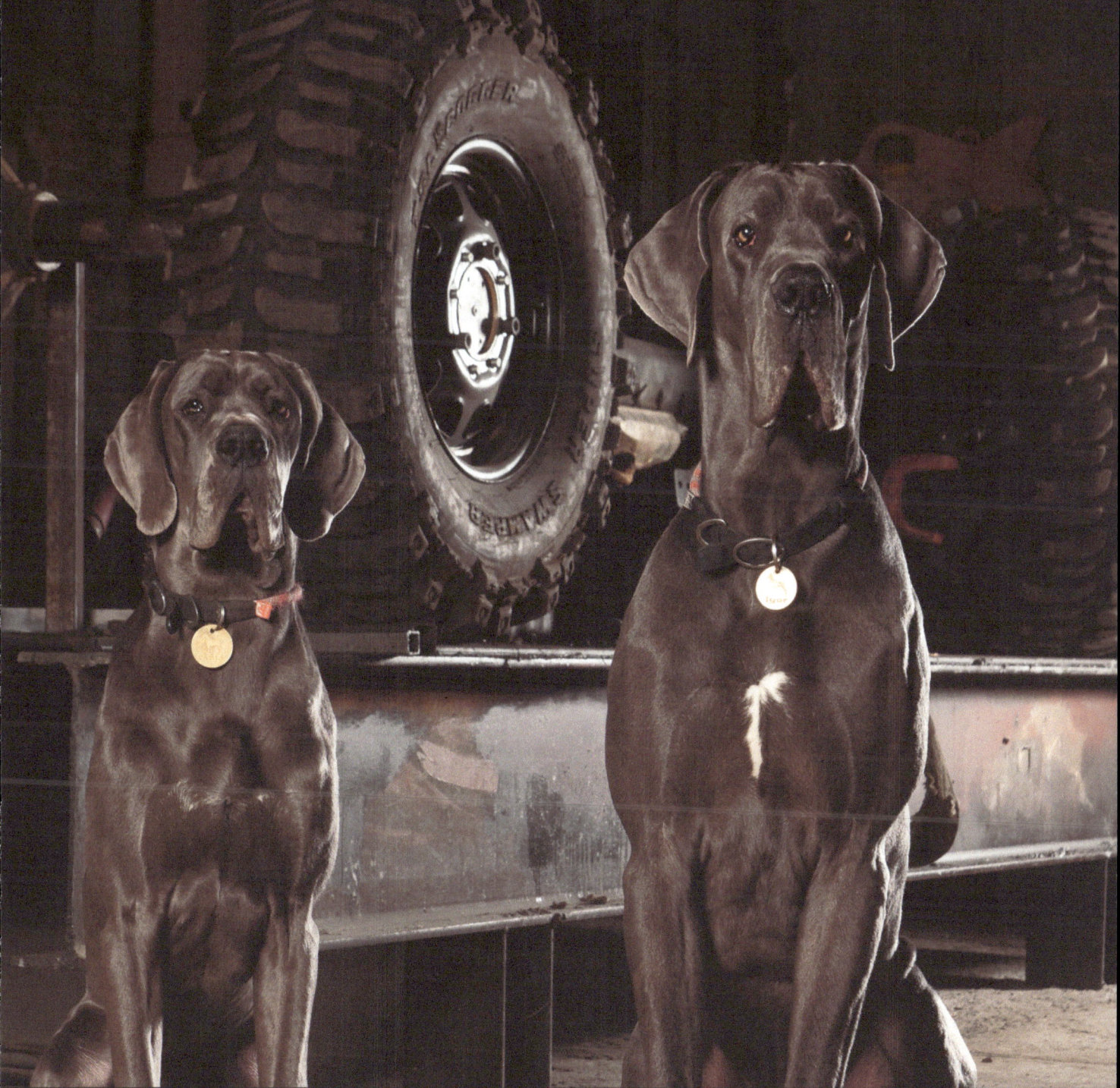

Great Dane

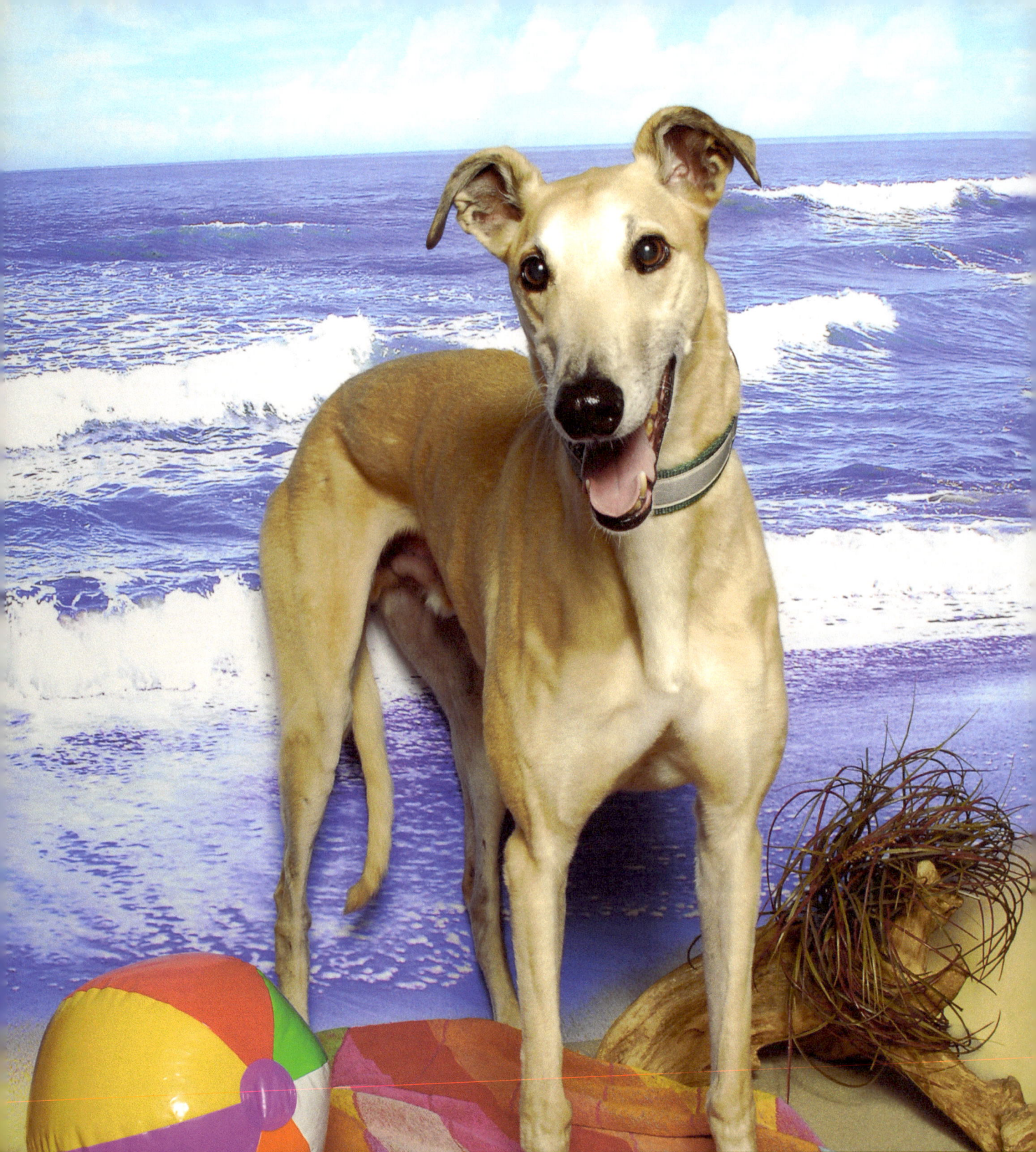

Greyhound

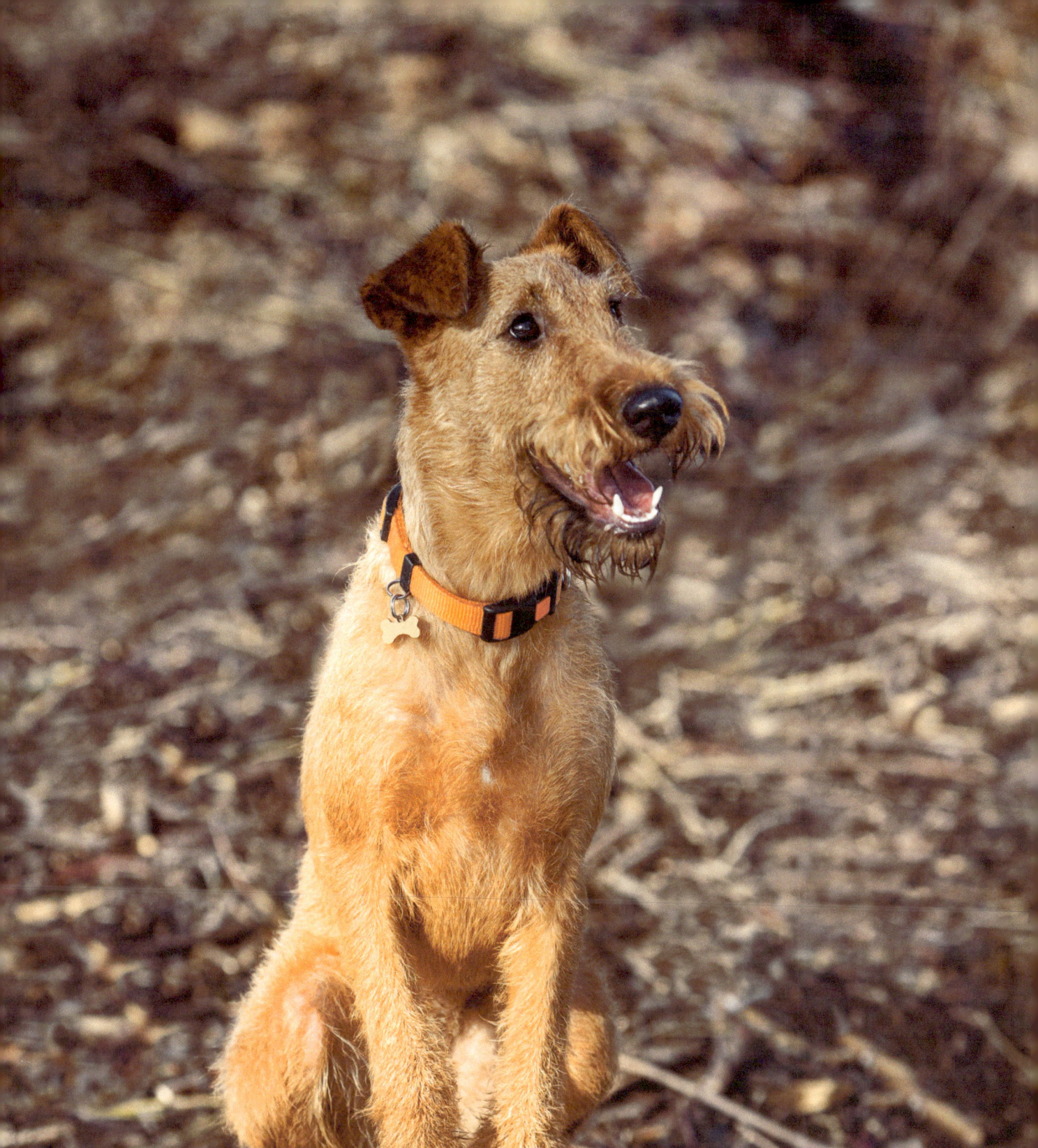

Irish Terrier

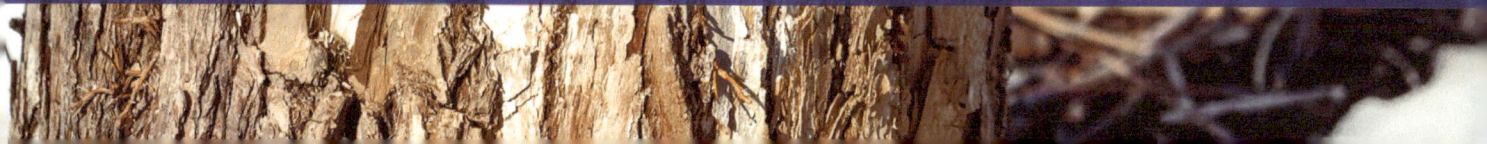

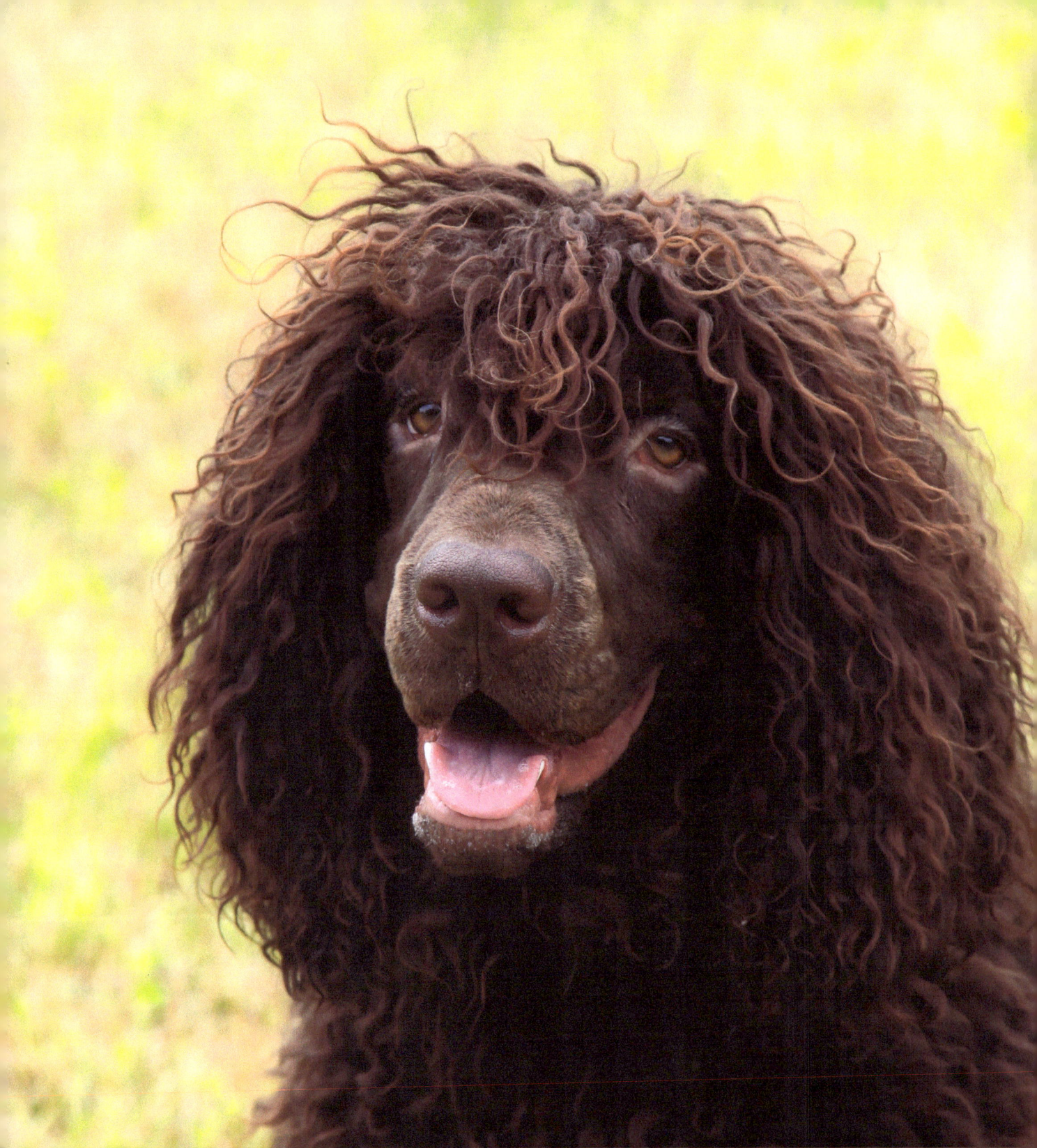

Irish
Water Spaniel

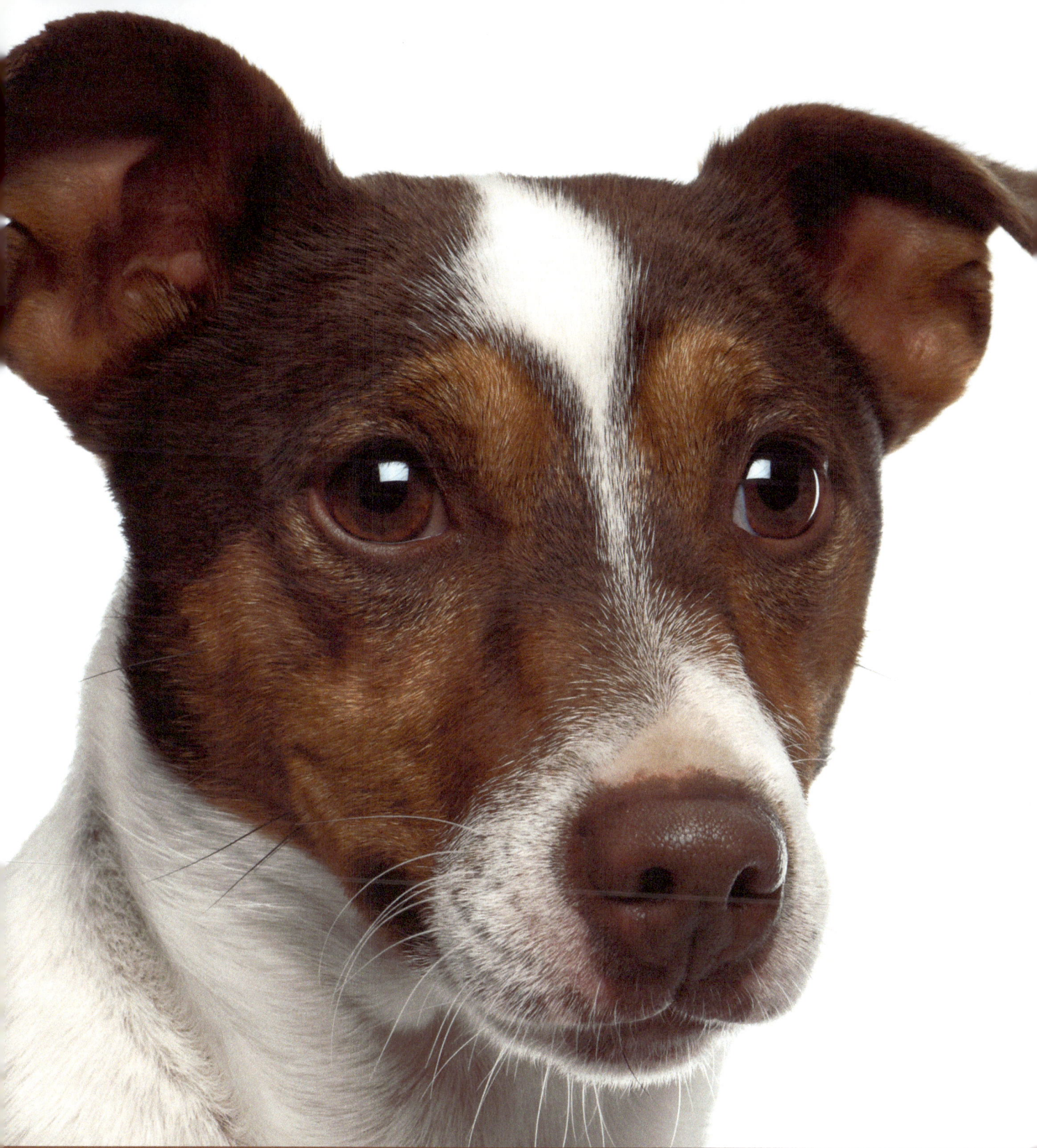

Jack Russell

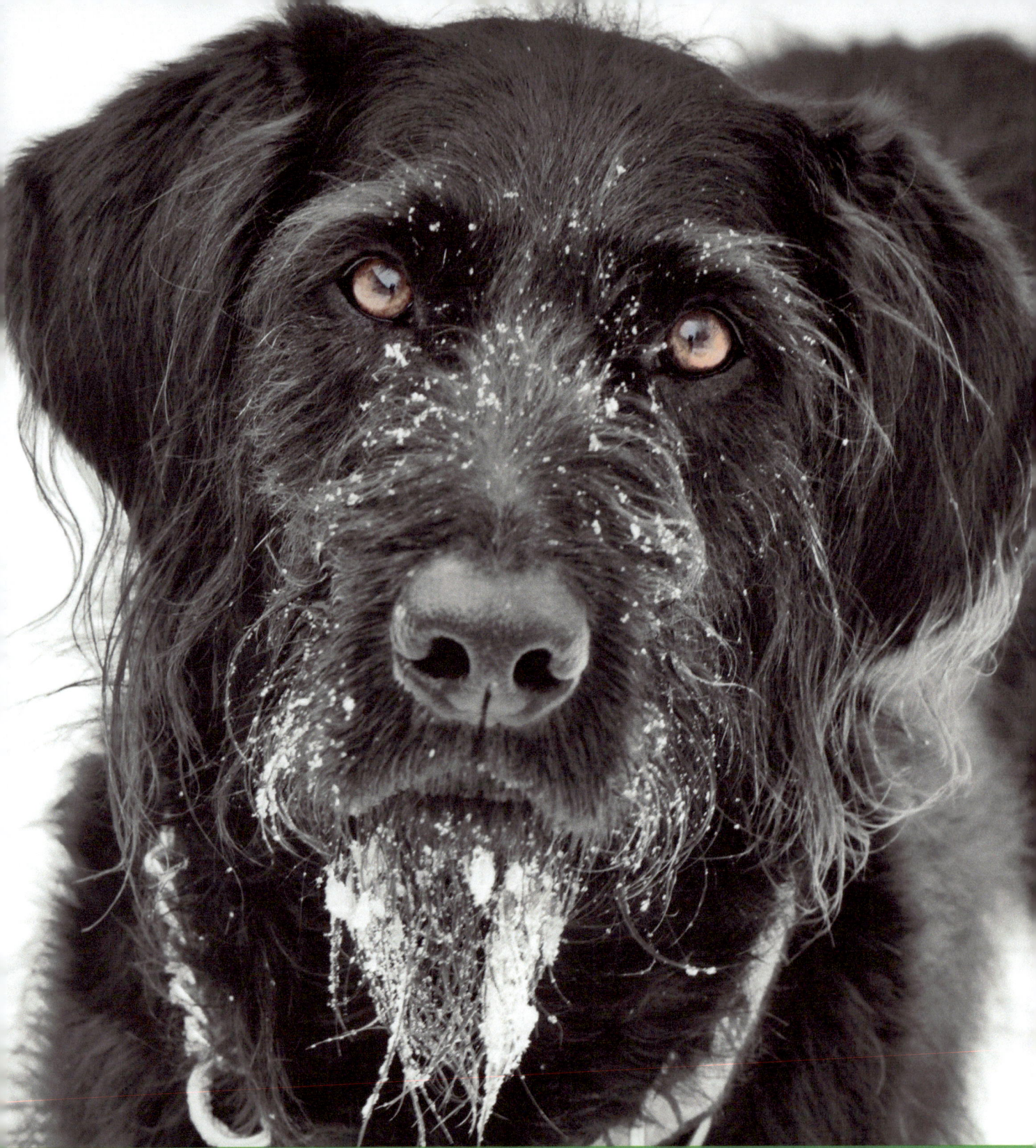

Labradoodle

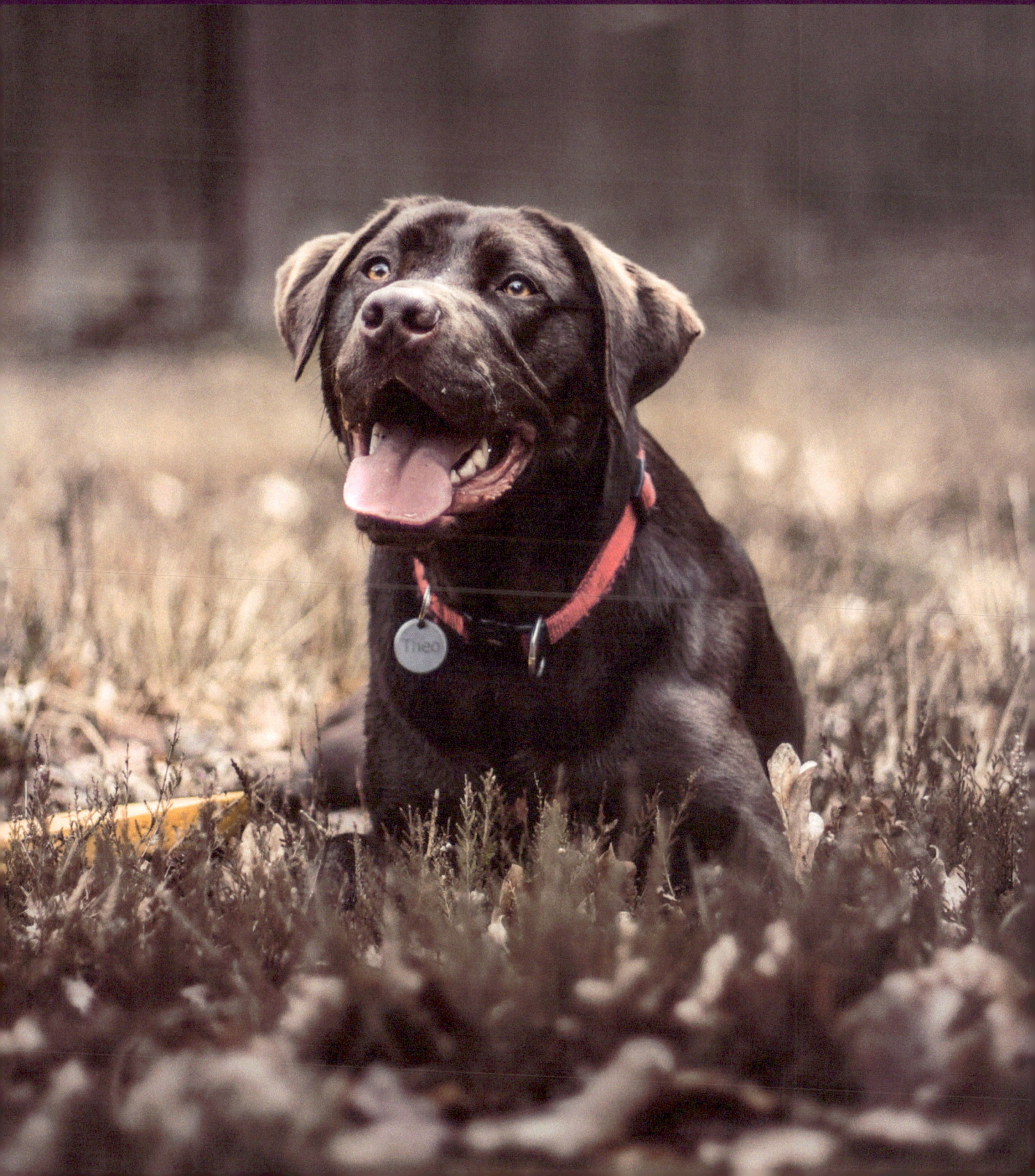

Labrador

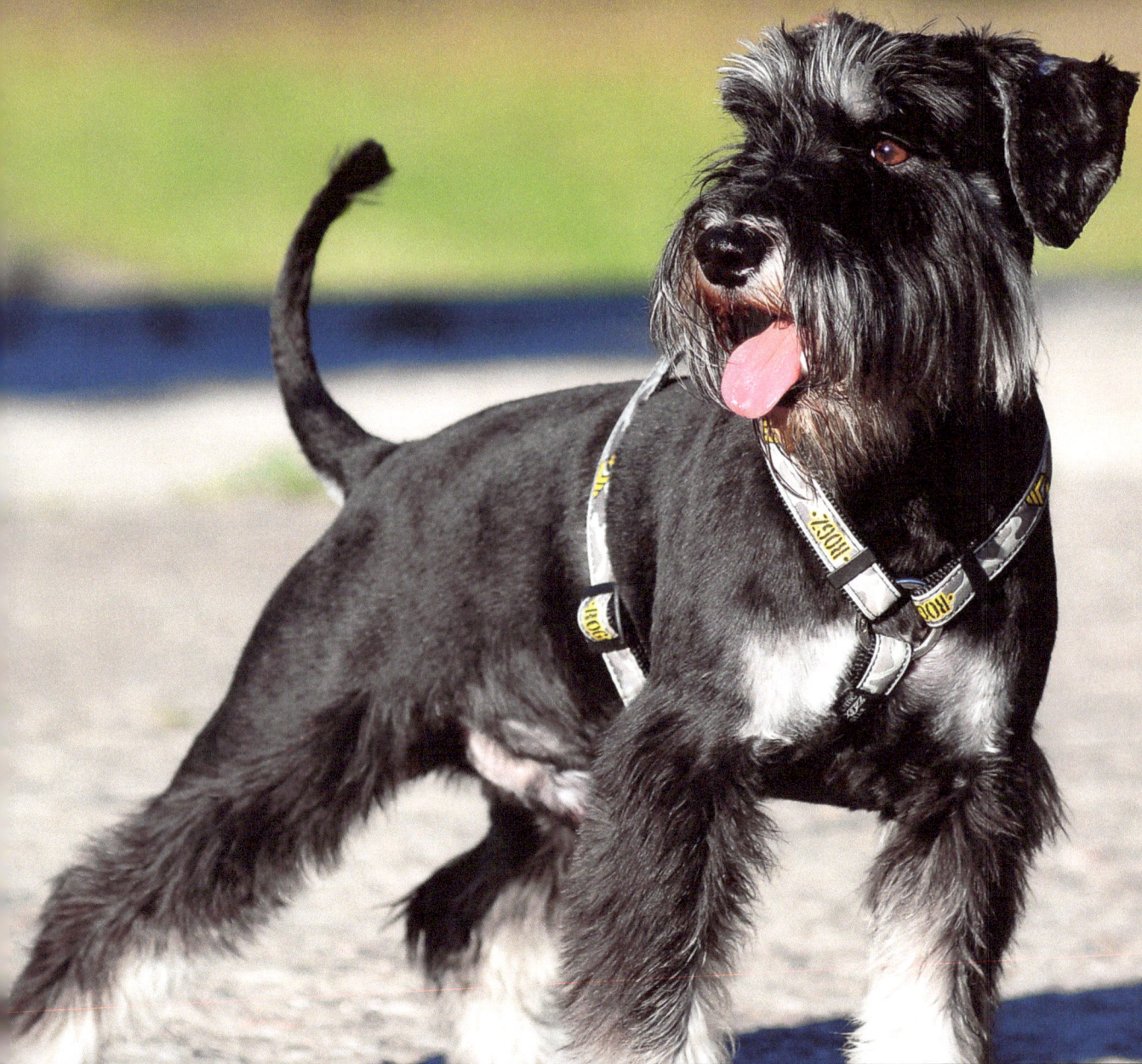

Miniature Schnauzer

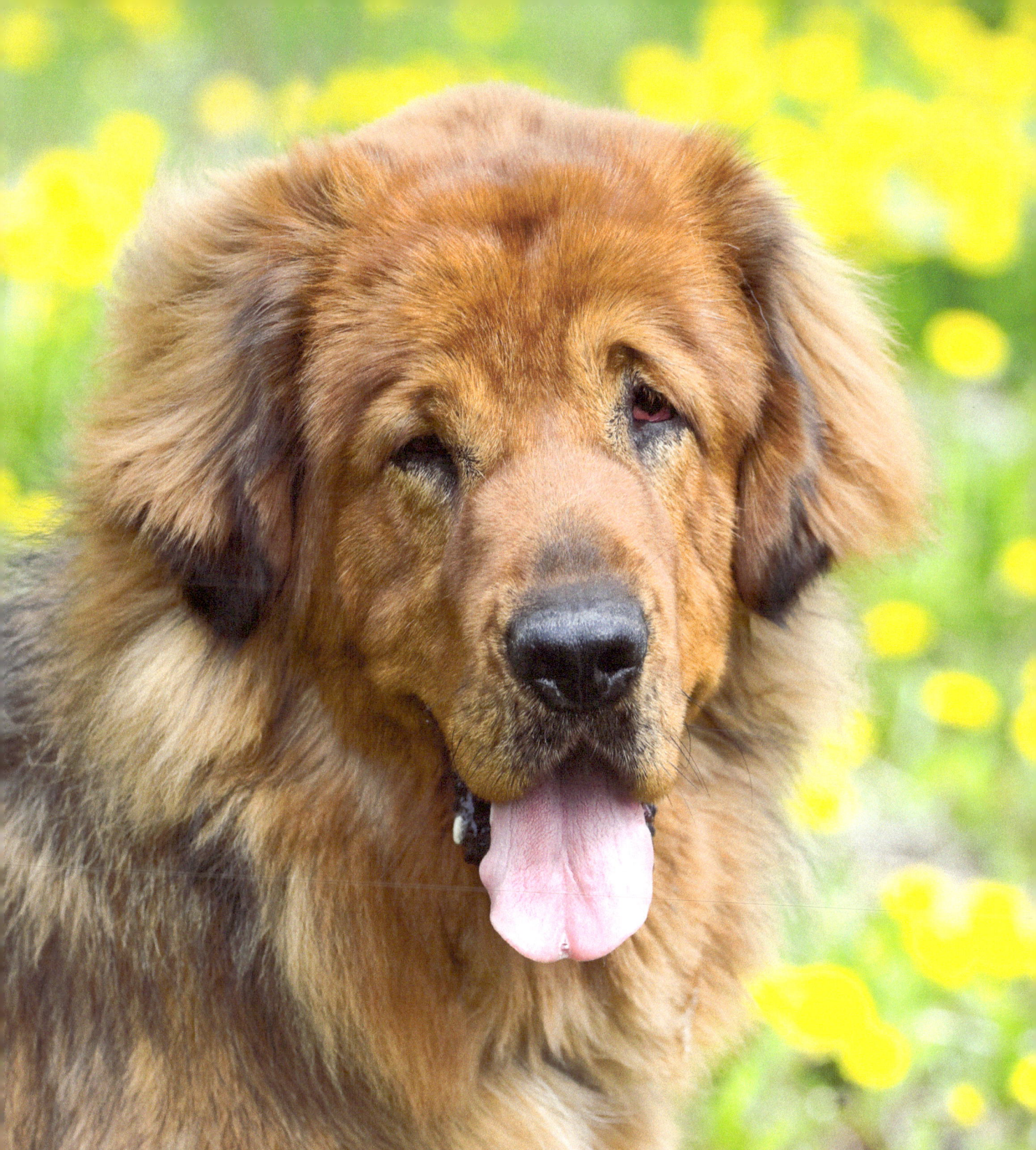

Newfoundland

Old English Sheepdog

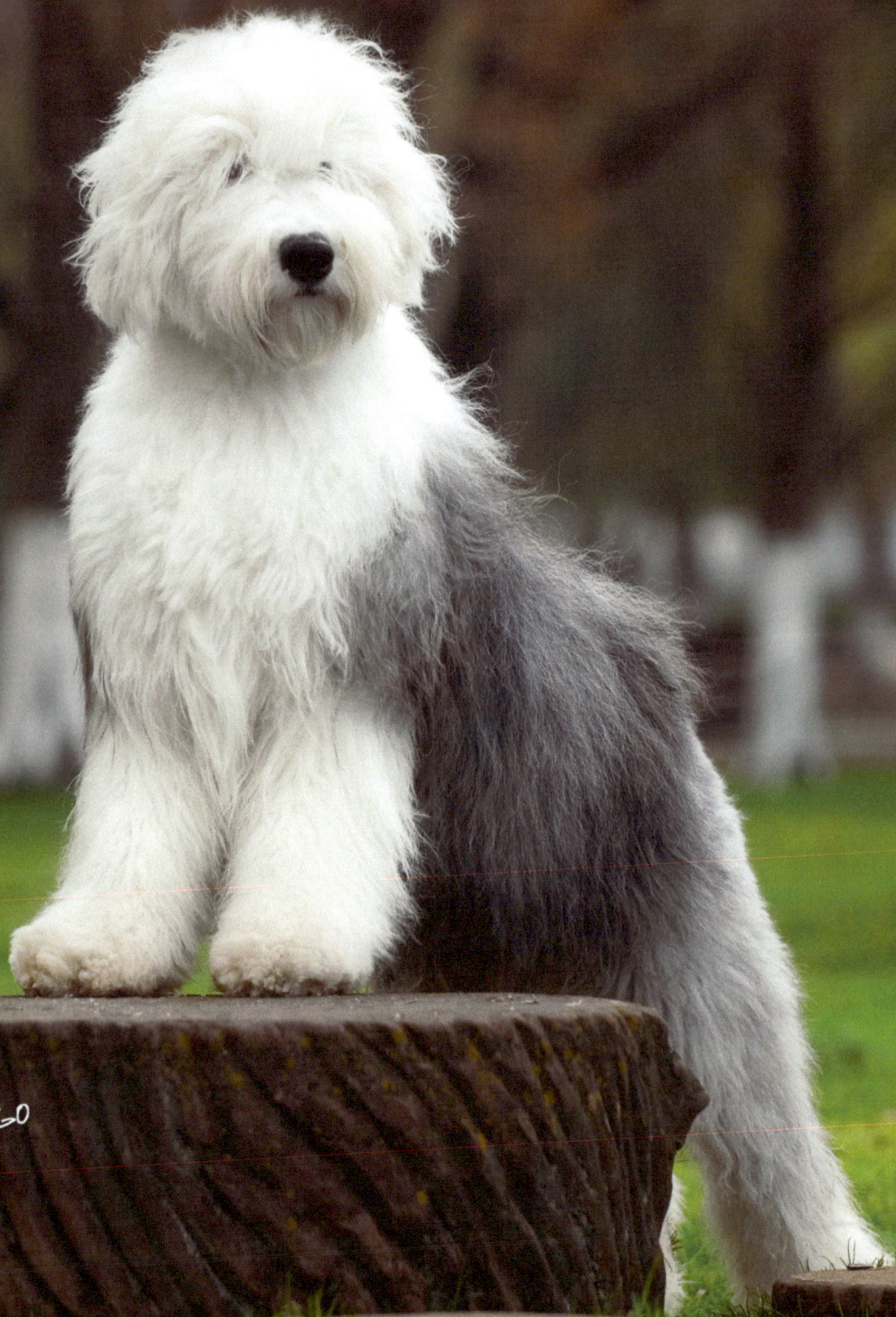

Pekingese

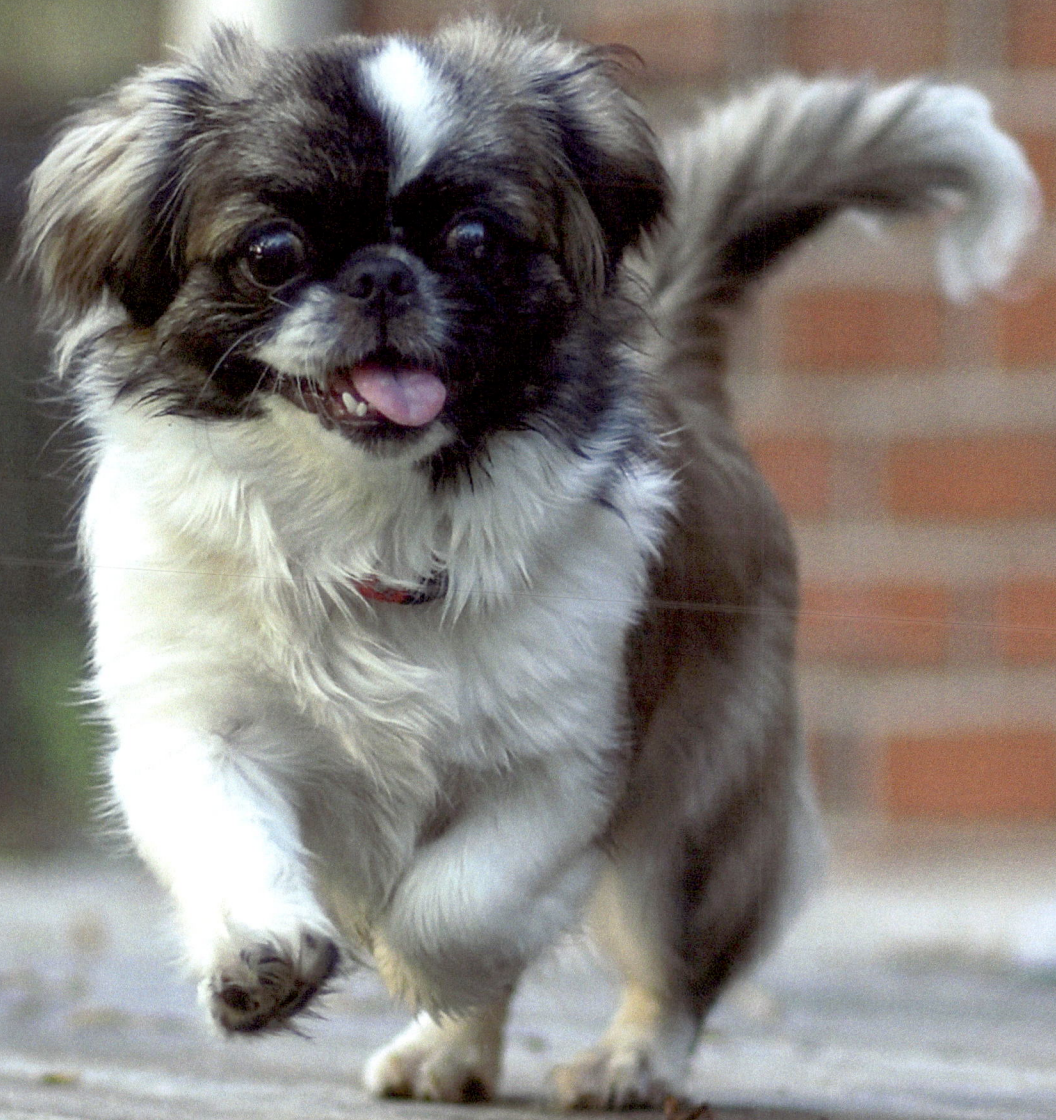

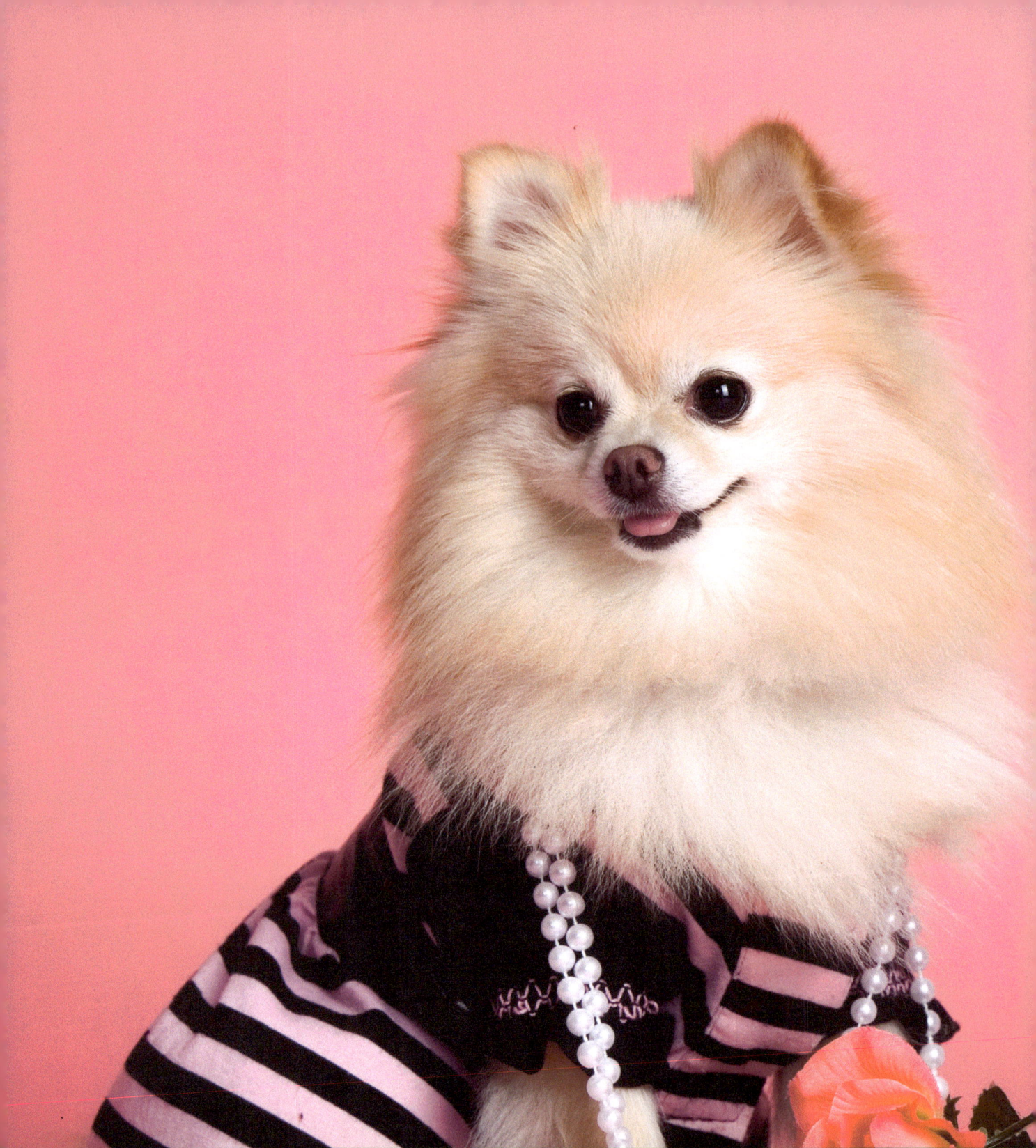

Pomeranian

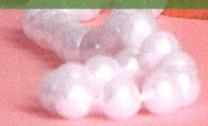

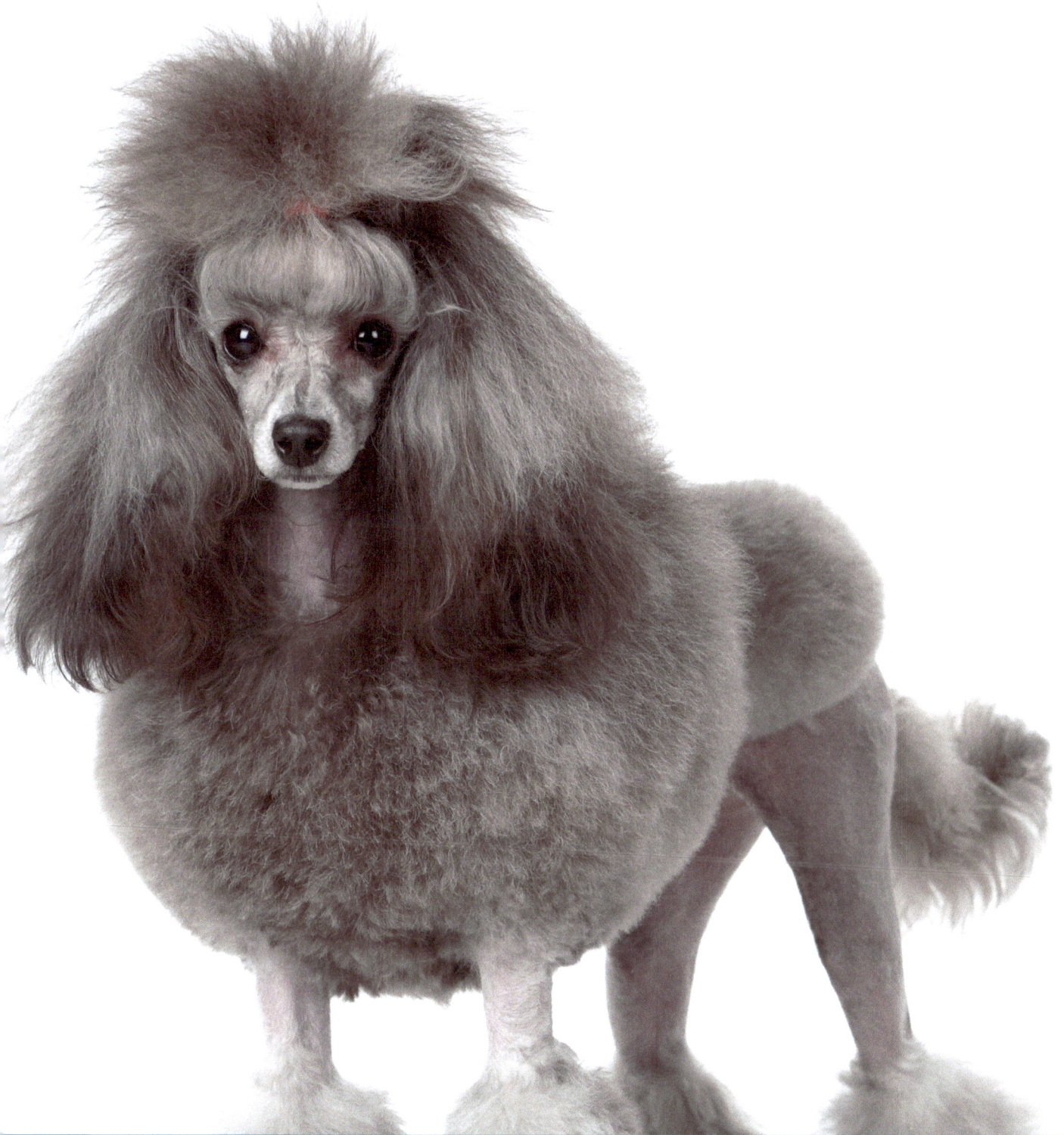

Poodle

Pug

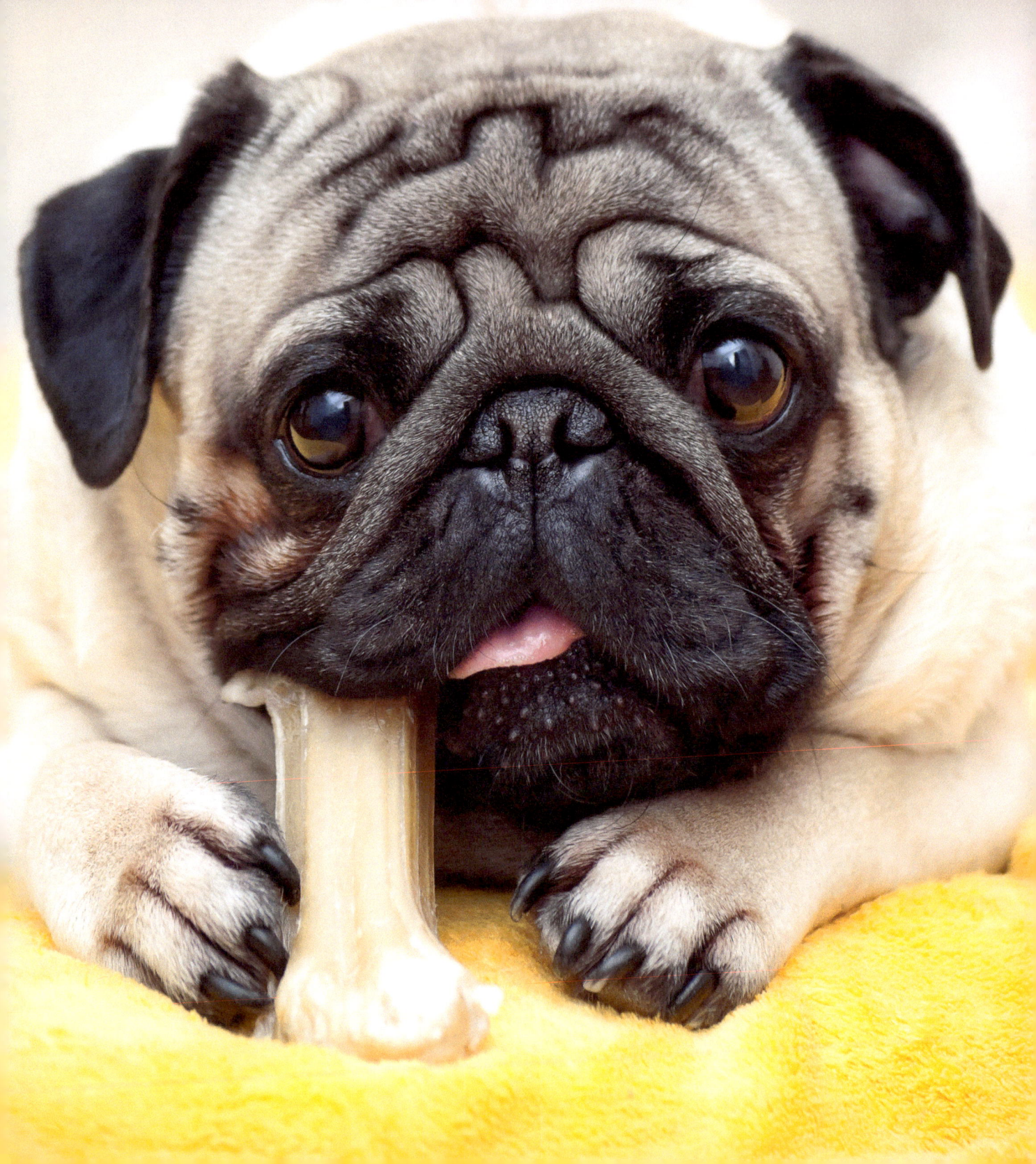

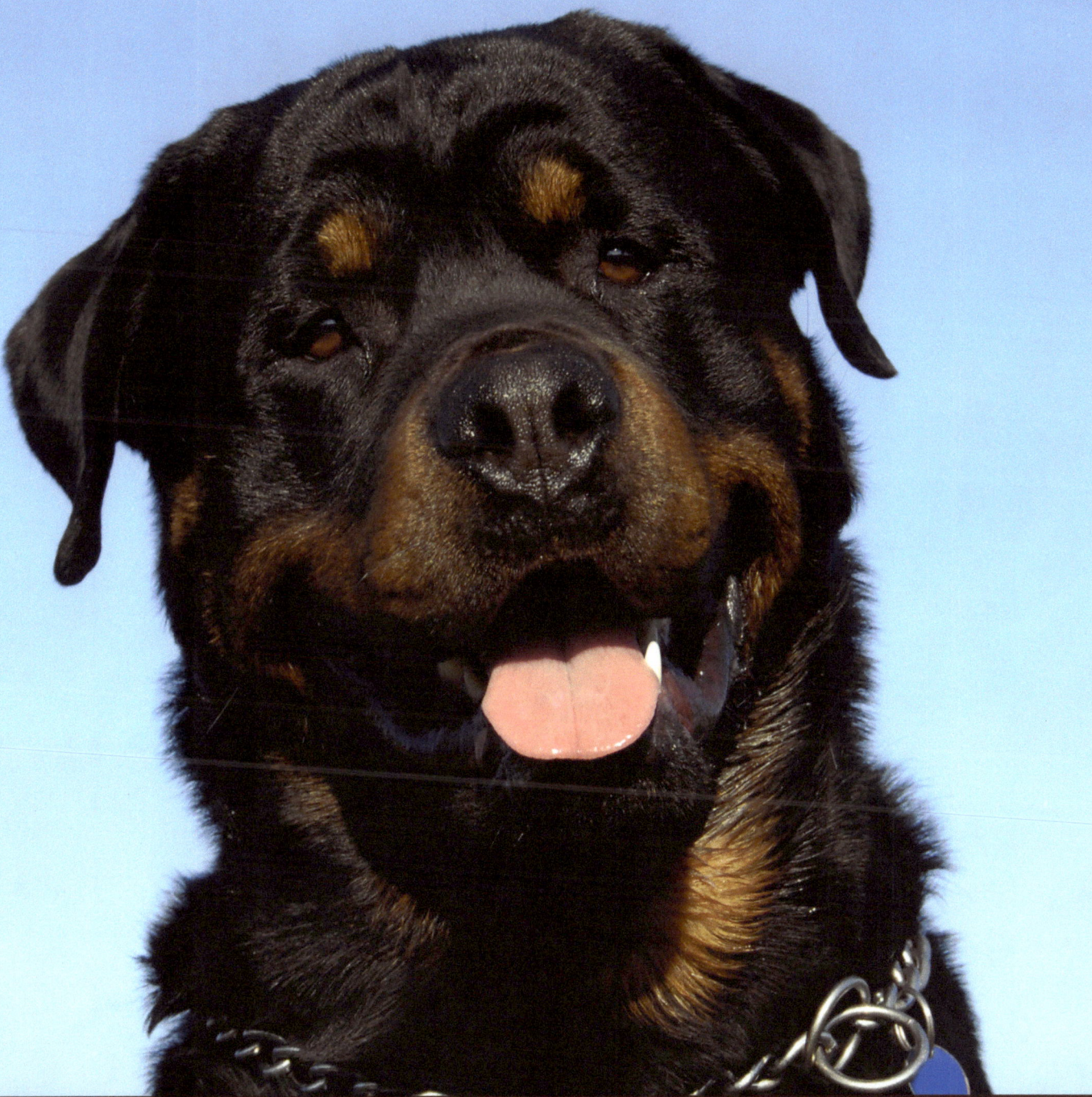

Rottweiler

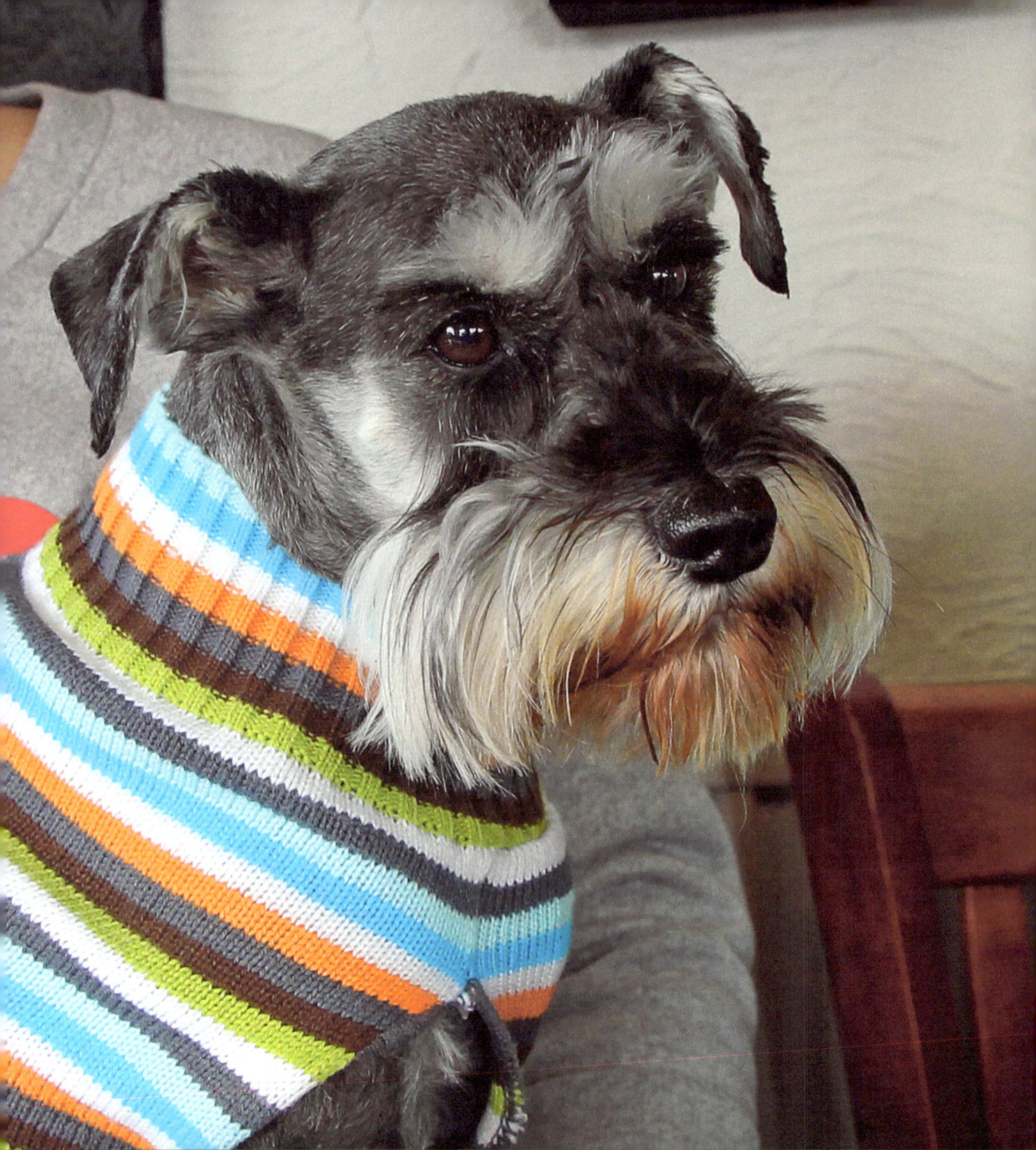

Schnauzer

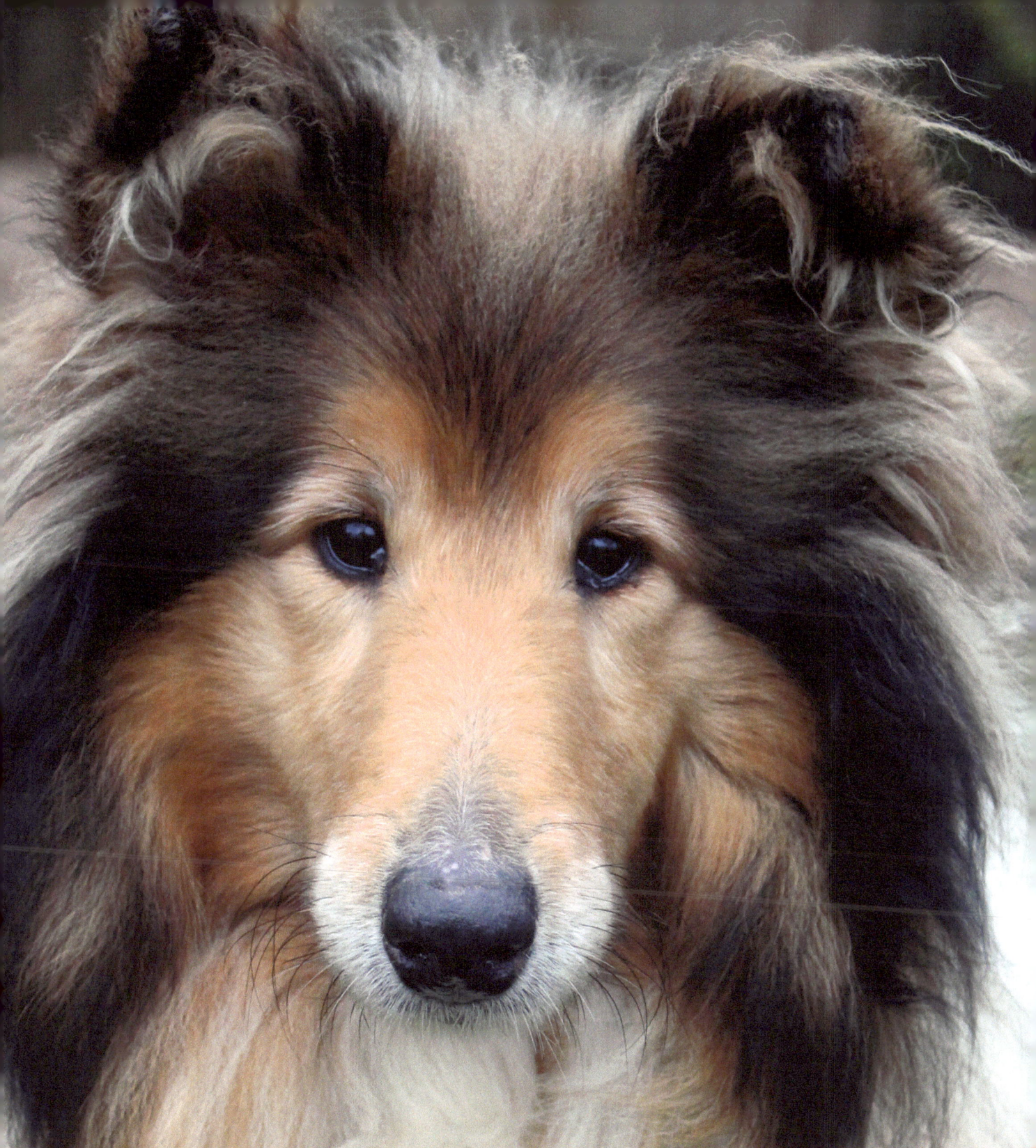

Shetland Sheepdog

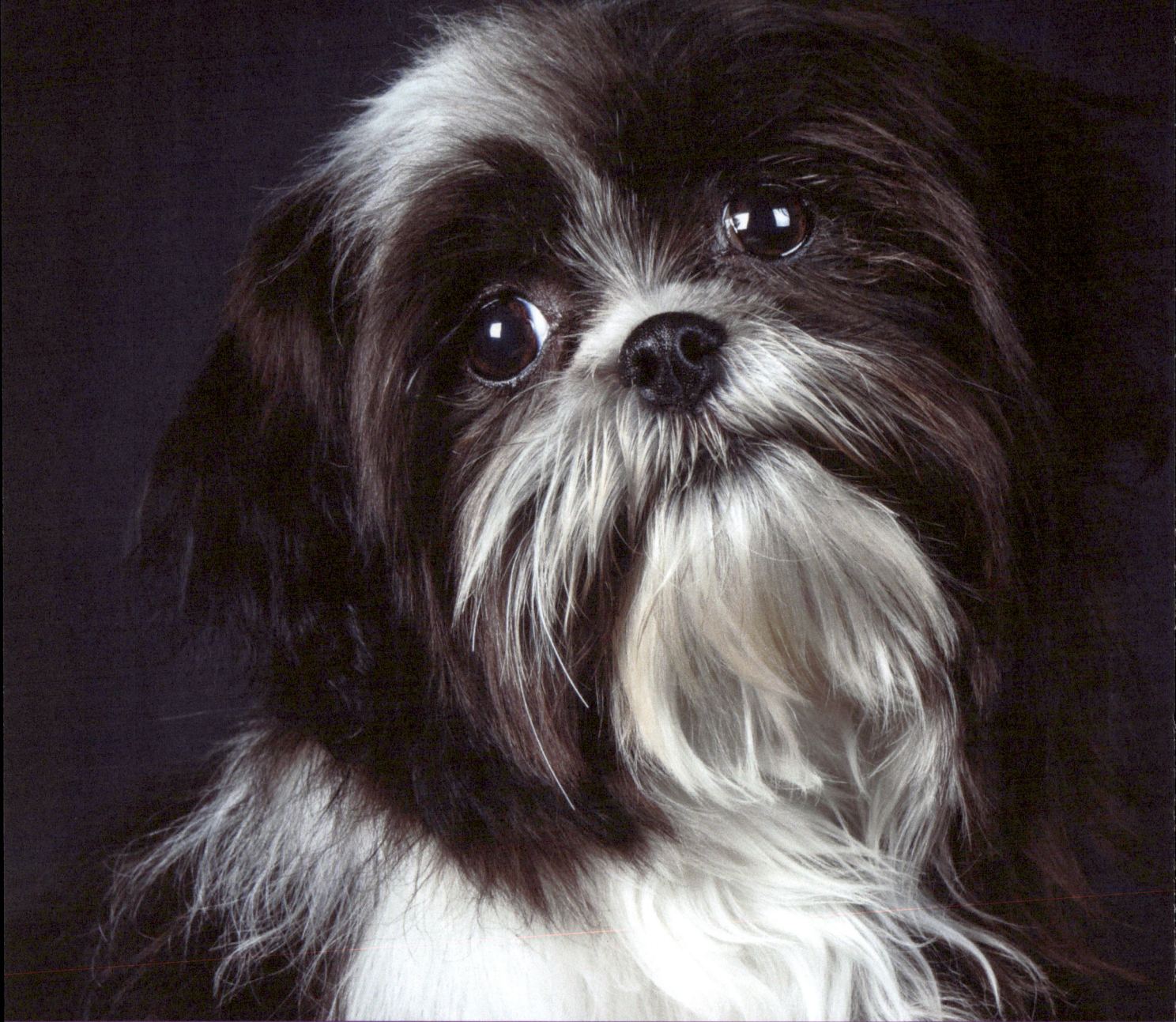

Shih Tzu

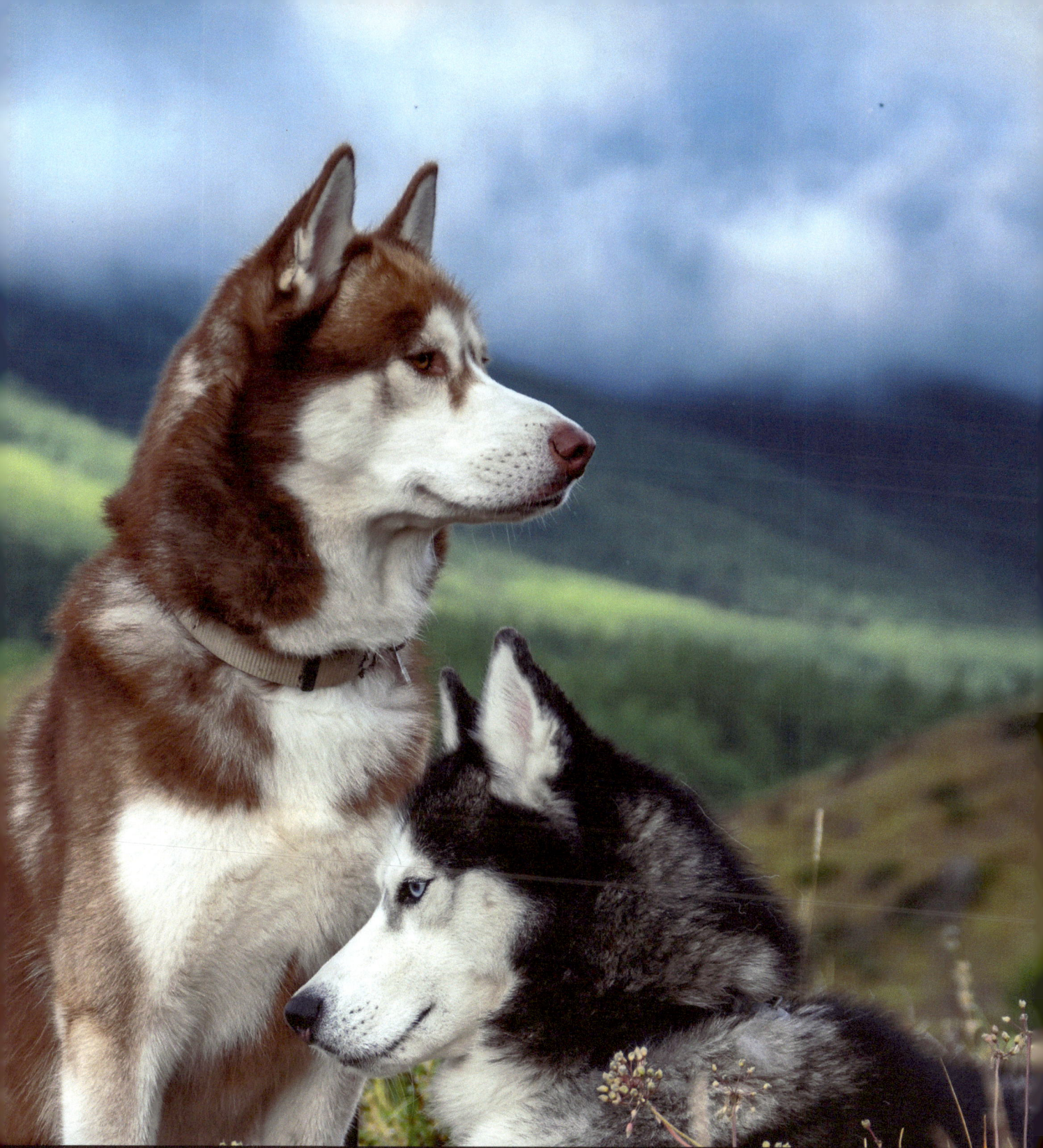

Siberian Husky

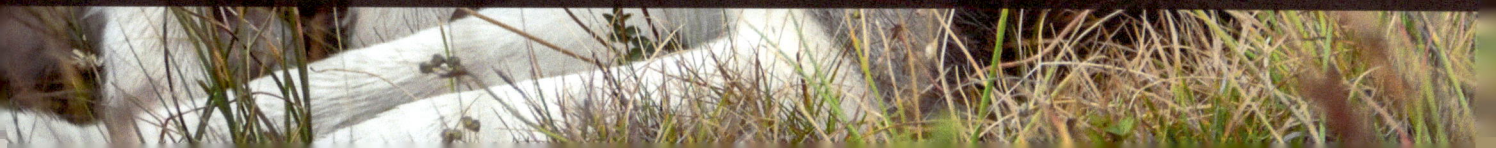

Springer Spaniel

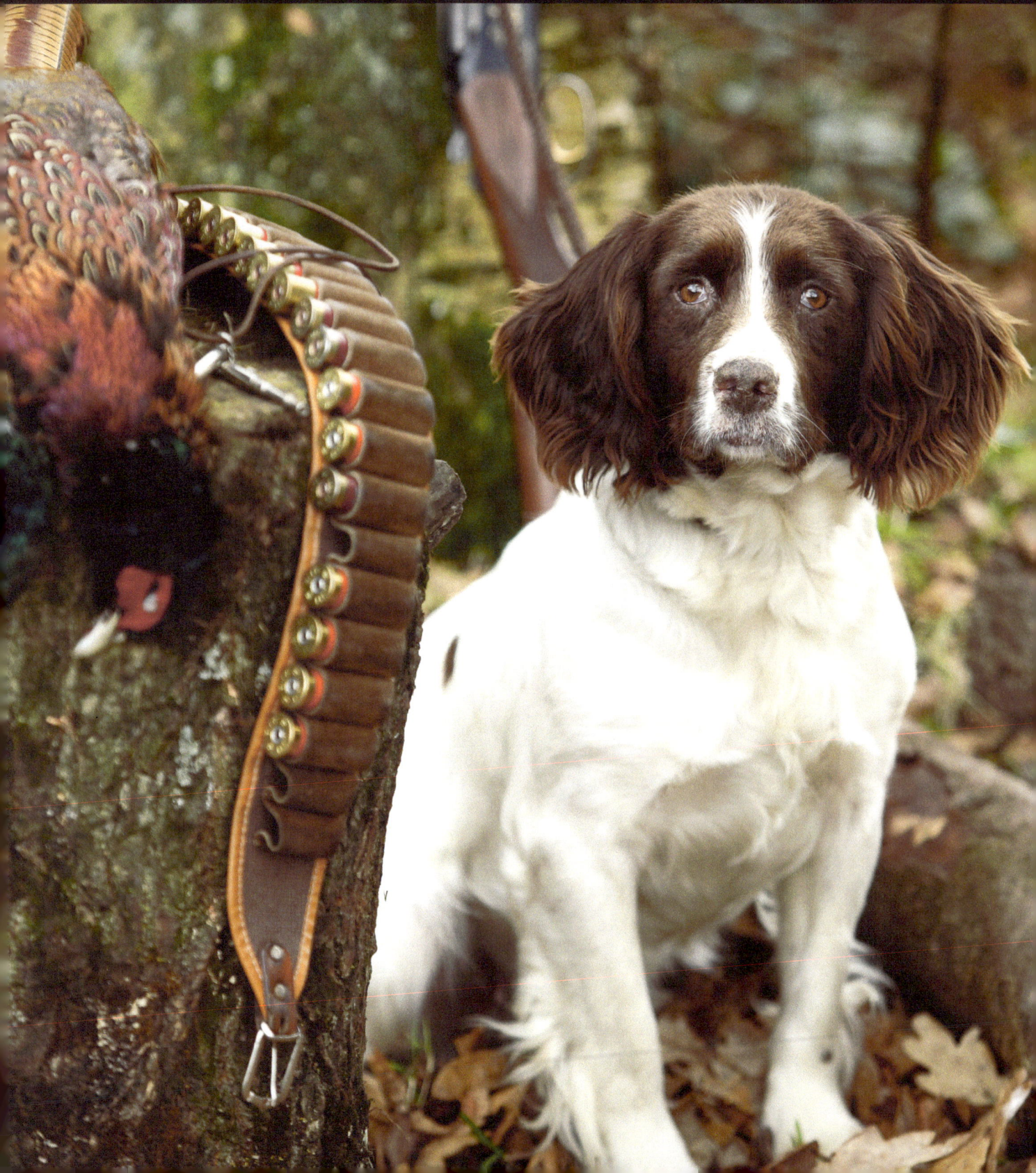

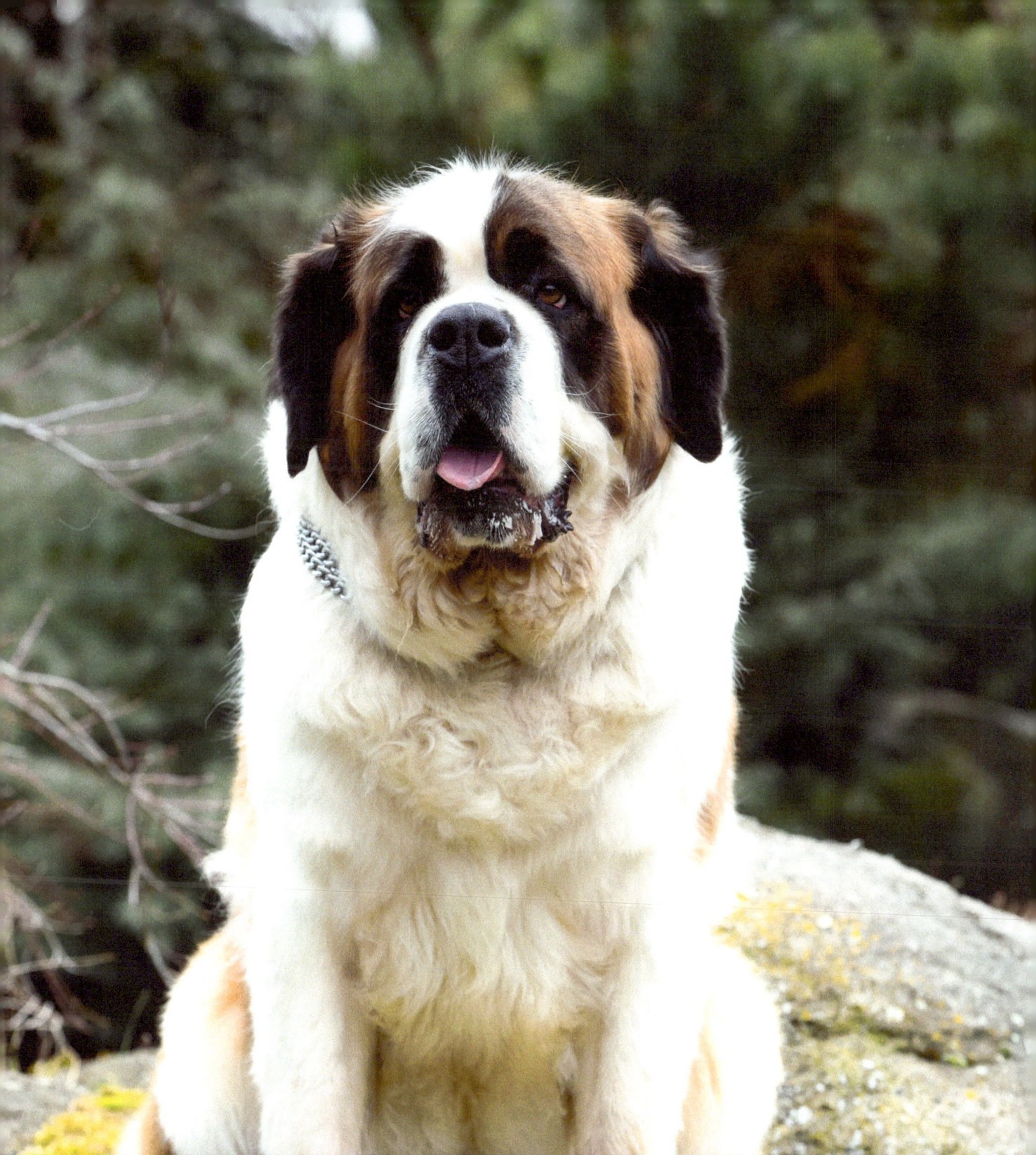

St Bernard

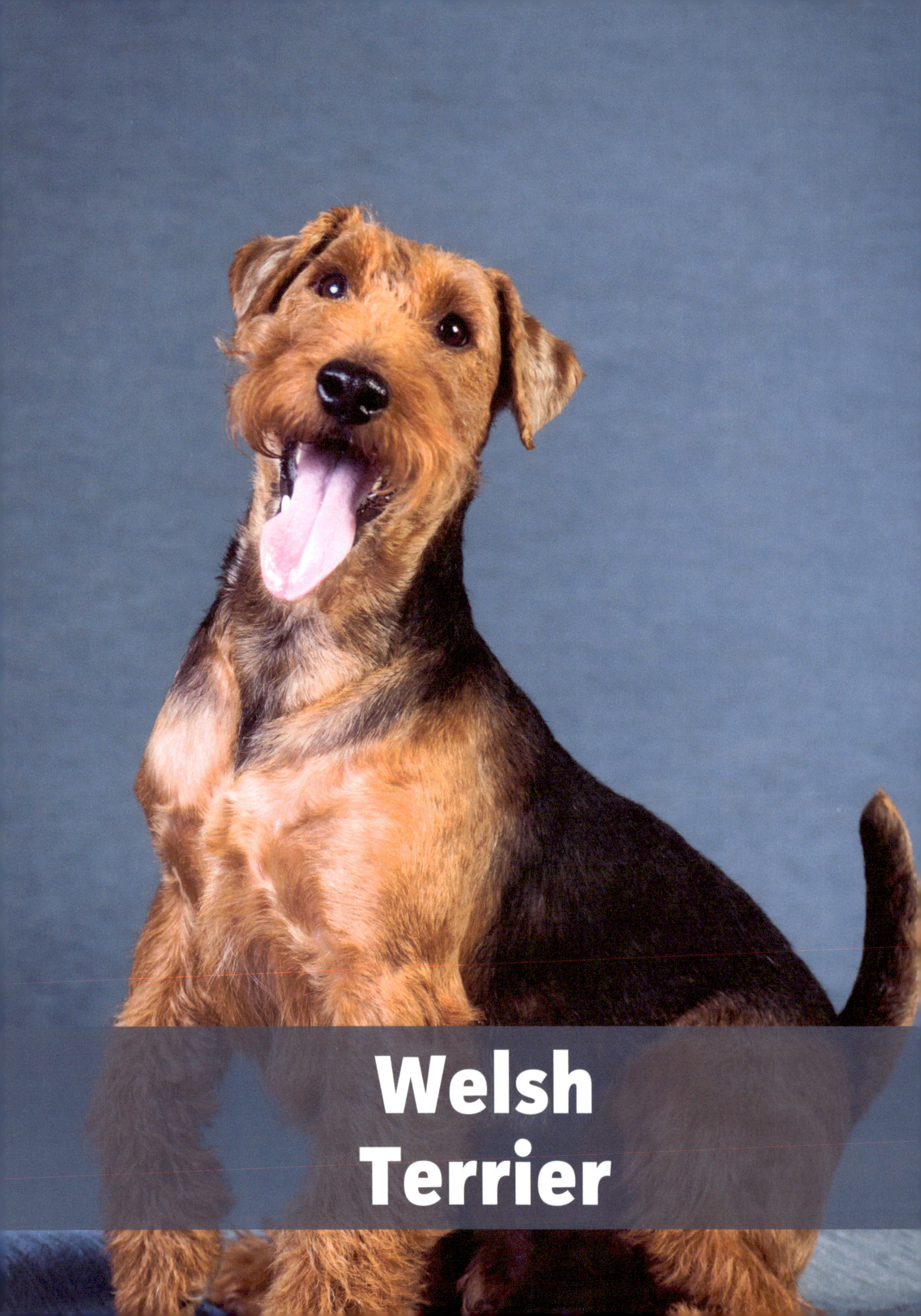

Welsh
Terrier

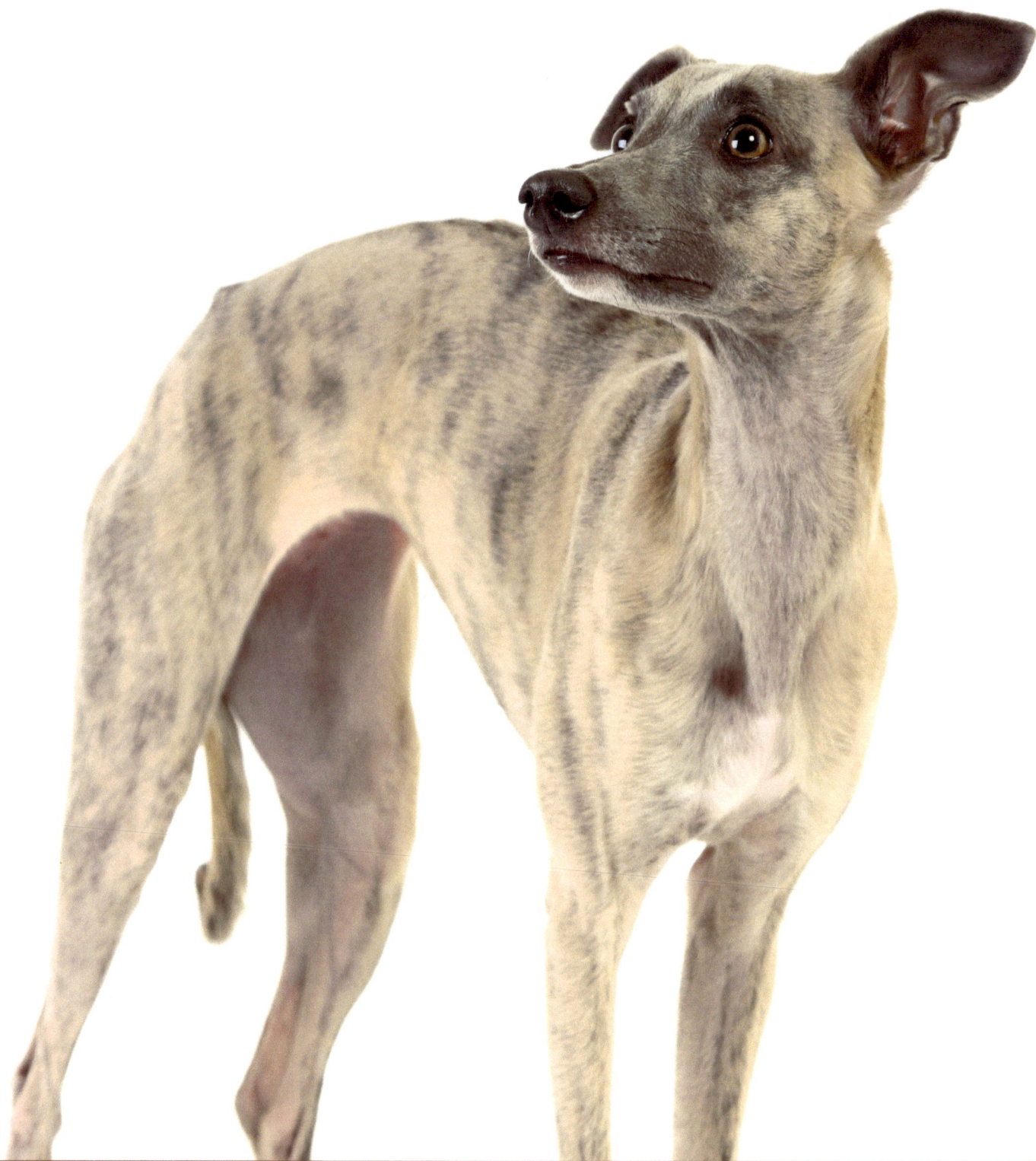

Whippet

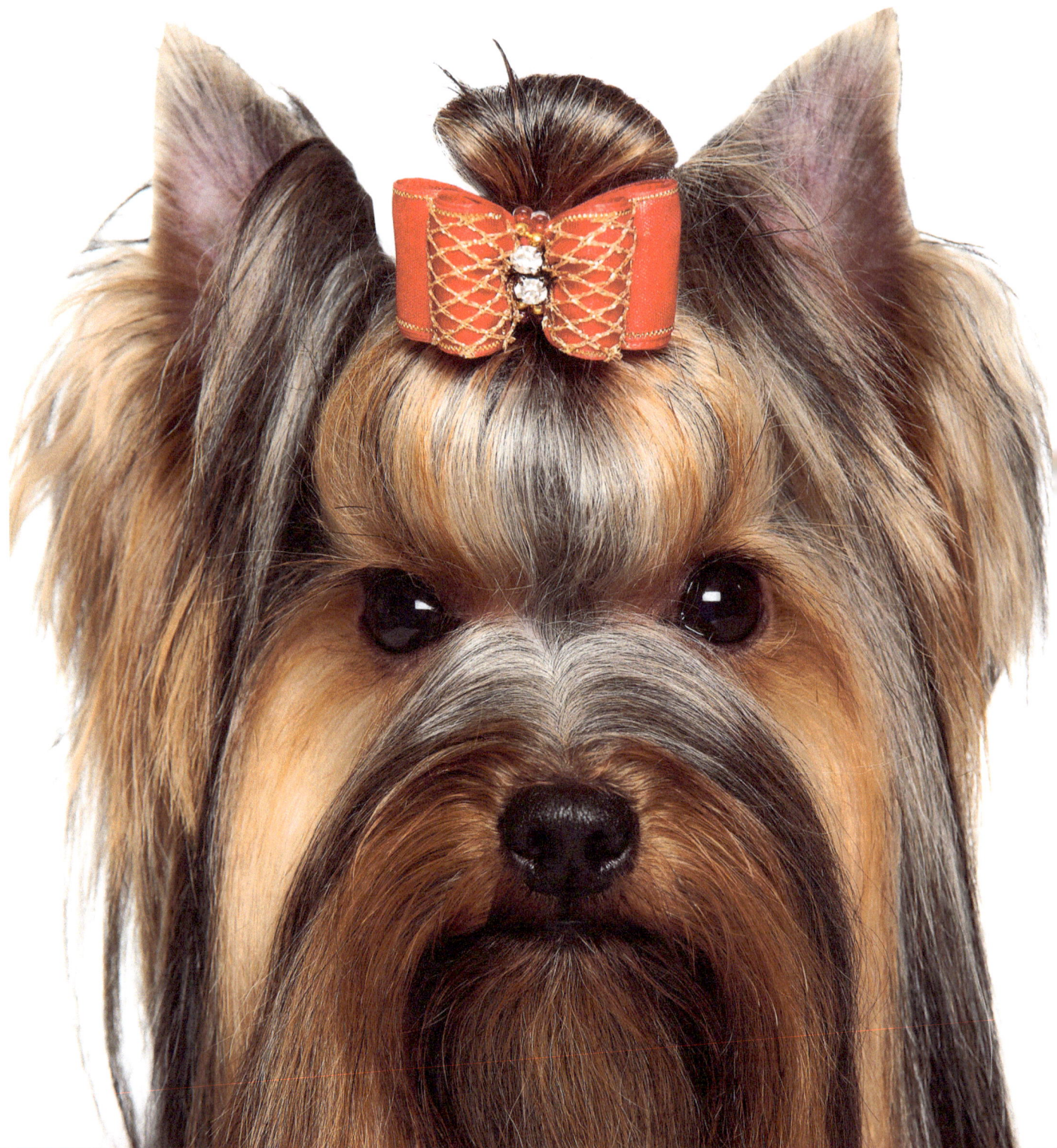

Yorkshire Terrier